Forever Loved

D1601578

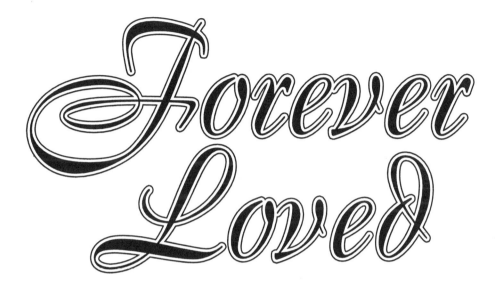

A Personal Account of
Grief and Resurrection

Gary R. Habermas

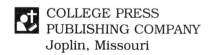

COLLEGE PRESS
PUBLISHING COMPANY
Joplin, Missouri

Library of Congress Cataloging-in-Publication Data

Habermas, Gary R.
    Forever loved: a personal account of grief and resurrection /
Gary R. Habermas
        p.   cm.
    Includes bibliographical references (p. 140).
    ISBN 0-89900-796-1 (pbk.)
    1. Habermas, Gary R.   2. Bereavement—Religious aspects—
Christianity.   3. Habermas, Deborah Ellen Chapman, d. 1995—
Death and burial.   4. Death—Religious aspects—Christianity.
5. Ovaries—Cancer—Patients—Virginia—Biography.   6. Christian
biography—United States.   I. Title
BR1725.H15A3 1997
248.8'66'092—dc21   96-29446
    [B]   CIP

With All of My Love,

To Robbie, Michelle,
Holly, and Kevin

In Whom I See
Debbie's Reflection

Table of Contents

$\mathcal{P}$rologue

As children, we were as different as night and day—but we were sisters. She was fair. I was dark. She was short. I was not short. She wanted to wrap her arms and legs around me like an octopus while we shared the same small bed. I wanted my space, wishing for a "board of nails between us" while we slept. She was a gentle spirit—Dad's "love bug." I was a rebel—Dad's "worry-wart." But we were sisters.

As teenagers, our family life crumbled with our parents' divorce. I became more rebellious. Deb became my defense attorney, trying to save me from my mother's wrath. Loving and serving the Lord seemed to come easy for Deb. I struggled with my faith, wanting to try what the world had to offer. But we were sisters.

As young adults, Deb married a Godly man—a theology student. I married a man of the world—a Vietnam veteran. Deb was my bridesmaid. I was her bridesmaid.

My marriage was rocky, ending in divorce 13 years later. Deb's marriage flourished until her death 23 years later. But we were sisters.

As adults, I returned to school to become a nurse with two children to support. Deb was a "stay at home" mom with four children. She baby sat for extra money to help support me and my children during my nurses training. (Deb made me promise not to tell anyone because she was "storing up treasures in heaven.") I graduated and remarried a wonderful man and again Deb was my bridesmaid—because we were sisters.

In April of 1995, I received a call. Deb had cancer and needed surgery. I was a nurse. I rushed to her side to save her—to nurse her back to health—to try to repay all the love and support she had so freely given to me all those years—because we were sisters.

Debbie lived four short months after her surgery. She wanted to be at home with her family she loved so much, so I came and used the nursing skills she had helped me attain and fulfilled her last wish. My faith was now strong. I knew God loved Debbie and was in control of her life and her death. I knew God loved me and allowed me to be a support and comfort for her and her family during her last days on this earth. Deborah Ellen Chapman Habermas died at 1:06 a.m. on August 9, 1995 and I miss her desperately, but I praise God—because we were sisters.

Judi Hanney, Sister

Mother-in-law! I have always been uncomfortable with that name. It seems to imply love demanded by law or an entitlement to love. From the time I met Debbie 25 years ago, she had my heart. Perhaps because of her quiet, unassuming nature, perhaps because of her diminutive size, I always felt protective of her. Through most of these 25 years, we lived apart in distant states, seeing each other only a few times a year. The last six years of her life, we were blessed with an unusually close relationship.

A move to Lynchburg, VA in 1989 brought a closeness neither of us could have anticipated. We were in touch daily either by phone or in person. It didn't take long to realize we had everything in common. We thought alike, at times reading each other's minds. Sometimes I would laughingly ask her, "Are we the same person only divided into two people?" Then we would laugh. We laughed a *lot*. We laughed at problems, we laughed at ourselves, we laughed at *everything*—silly things—I miss the laughter.

We could be ourselves around each other. Neither of us demanded the slightest change in the other. We loved to say we had the same weaknesses and neither of us had any strengths—laugh again! Always the laughter.

Debbie was generous to everyone. She was a "giver." If someone voiced a desire for a particular item, more often than not Debbie bought it for them out of her babysitting money. She helped relatives in need from time to time who never knew it was Debbie who gave to them. We liked to joke about what her responsibility to me would be when it came my time to depart this world. It was always accompanied by laughter.

Little did either of us know it would be Debbie leaving me instead of me leaving her. Even when she was so ill, she thought of my well being. When I would be changing her feeding tubes or giving her medications or doing any of the routines each day required, she would say, "Mom, I don't want you to take care of me and do all the work—you'll hurt your back." My back?? As if that mattered now! There was no more laughter.

Earlier I said Debbie was a "giver." Even in her last days and weeks, she gave us all the greatest gift. One that will remain with each of us forever. She demonstrated dying grace. I am thankful that all of our families who are scattered across this country could come to visit and to help with Debbie's care. So many witnessed the beauty of her praise to God with uplifted hands as she listened to her praise songs. She was a living testimony of her love to her heavenly Father and of His love to her. We look forward to that precious reunion in heaven where we will once again laugh—where I'm sure, when I arrive, she will introduce me to all the pleasures she presently enjoys. Together, we shall praise God and know then why Debbie went first.

Forever Loved is our best memory of Debbie, who was my daughter, my sister, and my friend.

Roberta Habermas, Mother-in-law

My experience with grief, the death of my little sister.

I was never really close to my little sister until after she was married and started her family. It was probably because I was married (far from home), and she was dating and going through those younger stages of life. My sister, Judi, was closer to her in age and they were very close.

After Deb's marriage, I would see Debbie when they came up for her visits with family. We grew close and I loved her dearly. She always impressed me with her quiet Christian demeanor.

When I heard of Debbie's cancer it stunned me and sent me into the presence of my Lord of Hosts, the one who is my God, who fights my battles. What did His Word say about healing? I wanted to support my sister in the best way I could, with His Word, and to encourage her and help her stay focused on Him. Her spirit had to be centered on Him, and not the cancer.

I know my "God is able to do exceedingly abundantly above all I ask or think." God never gives us more than we can handle and even prepares those He loves for hard times. At the time, I was doing a Bible study on the character of God. God is good; everything He does is out of love. He never gives us seconds (second best), only absolute best. I didn't have to understand, just believe.

Judi and I decided to go down to Virginia to help Debbie. Judi is a nurse and certainly more medically qualified than I. So what could I do? I resolved to help with cooking and cleaning. Then God led me to have devotions with the kids. I felt Holly and Kevin needed to know that God is good. God is Sovereign, in control of everything that was happening. Nothing catches Him off guard.

Every morning after the kids got up, they would get their Bibles. Holly, Kevin, and Megan (Judi's little one) all joined in. We would have sword drills, find a Bible passage, read and explain if they could. It was fun for them and I would choose verses that I felt would comfort and prepare them in the event that God would take their Mom home. God does love Holly and Kevin, even if He took their mother. Some good would come from these hard times. God knows all about us—our beginnings and our endings. He uses hard times to bring us into maturity (God's platforms to show us His strength) making us usable vessels for His Honor. God uses Christians who weather the storms of life in submission to His will. I don't believe He uses "hot house varieties" who are protected and never go through trials. It is these hard times that build character, molding us into the image of our Lord.

Jehovah Shamma (God who is there) always sees. He doesn't sleep and is always active in our everyday life. He sees and understands, the balm of Gilead that causes healing to come.

I consider my sister's funeral an offering of praise and worship to the Loving Father, who loved her in life and her death, who is real and personal. I still grieve over her loss, even now, but I sorrow not as others who have no hope, for I know I will see her again in robes of linen pure and white—COMPLETE IN JESUS.

Lynn Alexander, Sister

Have this attitude in yourselves which was also in Christ Jesus, who, although He existed in the form of God, did not regard equality with God a thing to be grasped but emptied Himself, taking the form of a bond-servant, and being made in the likeness of men. And being found in the appearance as a man, He humbled Himself by becoming obedient to the point of death, even death on a cross (Philippians 2:5-8, NASB).

1

Shock!

One of the attending physicians looked me in the eye and responded to my question: "I'm sorry, but I think your wife has ovarian cancer."

I wanted to scream: "Why her? She's only 43 years old!"

In that one second, my world had instantly changed. Fear clawed at my heart like I had never experienced it before. I could feel my stomach sloshing around inside me like water. I had to sit down . . . .

So that's what the doctor had meant minutes earlier, I thought to myself. After only a brief look at the sonogram image, he had said out loud, "You've got some serious problems here." At hearing the news, out of the corner of my eye, I had seen Debbie flinch. The gears were grinding inside me, too, but I didn't want to say anything in front of her. That's why I had asked the doctors to come out in the hall with me in the first place, a foreshadowing of the many times that would happen over the next few months. And now, this!

A barrage of unending questions immediately began to wage their assault. Was there a chance that the initial diagnosis was wrong? Could the shadowy images on the sonogram be incorrect? After all, the doctors had told me that other tests had to be run before a clear diagnosis could be made. Could it even be that Debbie's lifelong bout with colitis-like symptoms were causing these results? Should I consult a specialist? How many? Were any "miracle cures" available? What, if anything, should I tell my wife? On the other hand, how could I keep anything from her? Not only had we been totally open with each other all of our life together, but I was sure that my expression and emotions would give me away.

But there was a very different sort of question, too—and of an exceptionally painful sort. What about my four children, all of whom lived at home? Robbie was 21 years old, Michelle was turning 17 in about a month, Holly was 12, and Kevin had just turned 9. What effect would all of this have on them? **What** should I tell them? **How** could I tell them? But this line of questioning was too painful; I had to stop this! After all, we didn't know anything for sure. "Don't get the cart before the horse!"

Thankfully, my excruciating contemplations were interrupted. Shortly after the first doctor had given me his opinion, a second one had repeated the partial diagnosis about the ovarian cancer. But they had also made it clear that this was only a very early verdict—other tests were being ordered. Debbie was placed on a bed and I walked beside her as she was moved to a new location. I tried my best to maintain a "business as usual" expression.

Although she doubtless knew that something was wrong, I was not about to tell her the medical suspicions before the test results were more firm. I could still hope, couldn't I? Until then, I would have to bear my grim secret alone.

Deb was wheeled into a large, private room, awaiting the call for the additional tests. We were alone. I made sure she was comfortable. When she was resting and almost asleep, I mumbled something about letting my secretary know that I would not be in to teach my classes at the university. Just a few feet from her doorway, I found a telephone.

It was then that I first began to feel totally forlorn. Whom could I tell? Could I speak without Debbie overhearing me? But then again, how could I even talk on the phone? Battling back more emotion than I had ever before had to deal with, I called my secretary and cancelled the classes that were to begin in just a matter of minutes.

My next call went to my mother. What can one possibly say at a time such as this? "They think Debbie has cancer," I lamented. "I can't believe that she might be dying right now."

My mother was almost as shocked as I was—she and Debbie had always been very close. I imagine that she offered the advice we all expect from our parents: "Don't be so worried just yet. We don't know anything for sure." But whatever her words were, I don't remember them. There was one, and only one, solitary subject on my mind.

There were other phone calls that morning, sandwiched around trips into the room to see Debbie, who was yet to be wheeled away. Lying on her back, she was dozing, and I didn't want to disturb her. So back to the telephone I would go, hoping against reason that someone would share some useful information with me. Perhaps someone would even come rushing in at any moment and tell me that it was all a mistake.

I found myself reflecting on our shared past. Somehow, one phrase got lodged in my mind and was severely painful: Debbie was still my "little girl." I remembered well the first time I ever saw a picture of her. Her mother, with whom I worked, had shown it to me with the "challenge" that her daughter could "twist me around her finger." And oh, how good looking she was! I had had a picture in my mind for some time of what my perfect girlfriend would look like—and there she was! Was this a story-book fulfillment of the perfect love? Do those things happen in real life?

I met her a short time later. She was only 5'2" and 104 pounds, with green eyes and blondish-brown hair. I already thought that she was the "ideal" lady. Both of us were coming off of near-engagements. I met her on a Monday and asked her out the next day for a week-and-a-half in advance. She accepted and neither of us had ever dated anyone else again.

When we got engaged, I had wrapped her ring inside successively smaller boxes. As she got down to the last one, I leaned over and whispered in her ear, "Will you marry me?"

With a quizzical expression, she said, "Yes, but why are you asking me that?" Then she opened the last box and found out.

Now we were less than three months away from celebrating our twenty-third wedding anniversary together. . . .

"Hello," intoned my mother's voice on the other end of the receiver, shaking me out of my reverie.

I distinctly remember the sobering words coming from my lips: "Mom," I confessed, "Debbie's still my little girl. And I've already buried her 100 times."

Given my mother's never less-than-positive demeanor, I was staggered by her admission: "I know, I have, too," she wailed. Now I had my first chance to try to cheer someone else. I realized that many people could be affected by the outcome of these tests!

I went back in to be with my wife. Other memories from our past also intruded on my mind. Some of them were not welcome. Our last few months, for whatever reason, had been among our best. We had always been exceptionally close, but these were extraordinarily so. At one point, Debbie had given me two little stuffed animals—two hedgehogs, the male with a little bow tie and the female with a babushka. They were holding hands and smiling.

But other images were far more painful. I could not even bear to think about them at this time. The one that most ravaged (somehow this word is not even strong enough) my memories concerned another gift that Deb had given me just shortly before. It was a little figurine of two mice huddled together under a leaf that was wrapped securely around them. Although rain drops were dripping all over, they were dry and almost appeared drowsy, relaxed and leaning on each other. The female was dozing while the male had his paw around her shoulders.

I remember well Debbie's words when she gave me the gift. "This is how I've always thought about our marriage," was all she said. The words were so precious at the time and I hugged her to me for several moments. But oh, how touching this scene was to remember now! The scenario stung my mind much more surely than any bee could ever sting my body. To get halfway through this episode was simply to cry out in pain and anguish. I had told my mother that I wondered if I could ever look at the two little mice again.

And then there was the cross-stitch pattern that she had made for us and framed some years before. I had specifically picked out the pattern and message. A little male and female angel sat together on a cloud, with contented looks on their faces. Underneath were the words, "But love goes on forever." It had hung on the wall over our bed . . . .

The phone rang and the nurse came in to get me. I received a call from my close friend and former department head, Dave Beck. He had already heard the news back on campus and was intent on coming to the hospital to be with me. "I don't really want any visitors," I told him nicely.

"Well, I'm coming anyway," he informed me in his matter-of-fact manner. "You need someone and I want to be there for you."

Surely enough, he arrived shortly. Debbie was even more relaxed and I couldn't bear to have her overhear my conversation, so Dave and I walked a very short distance away and talked. I could still see her from where we stood. I don't remember what I told him, but given our natures, I'm sure we philosophized about the situation.

As we stood outdoors, only a few feet from the nurse's station, I noticed the first of many ironies. It was springtime, and the warm sunshine should have signified the re-emergence of life. But until I heard the final medical verdict, only the thought of death occupied my imagination.

Another paradox surfaced in my discussion with Dave. "You know, this is really strange," I began. In 1990 I wrote a book on the subject of doubt, followed by another volume on death and eternal life in 1992. And now, if the doctors are right, I may experience the last theme "up close and personal."

Dave then gave me a compliment that he was to repeat during the next few months. "I've been thinking about what you've gone through this morning," he began. "You're doing a lot better than I would be if I had gotten the information that you have been given." Somehow, that comment encouraged me. It had perhaps been two hours since the ordeal began and, for the first time, I felt just slightly in control of myself.

While Dave and I were talking, two ministers arrived from my church. I was both amused that word traveled so quickly and glad to see friends, although I still remember saying quietly to Dave before I even recognized the visitors: "Oh, no. I sure hope this isn't so-and-so." I wanted to be left alone, but was a bit afraid of my own thoughts. As Dave had said, I did need friends there with me, but I don't think I recognized it at the time. These were the first of many contradictions, ironies, and mixed emotions.

Minutes later, Jerry Falwell also arrived. After looking in on my wife from a little distance away and offering some comforting words, the ministers left. Promising to be back after fulfilling an appointment, Dave also left.

When the others had been present, I had repeatedly excused myself and walked the few feet to see how Debbie was feeling. Now I returned to the room and awaited the testing. Pacing was the order of the day. After being told to drink a foul-tasting liquid (and not getting much of it down), she was taken away to have a CAT scan. I went with her, hoping to be able to stay with her the entire time. We had always been inseparable, so why should this be any different? But I ended up waiting in an adjoining room.

What was to happen here was the most meaningful single event of the next few months. I will never forget what transpired during the next hour.

While sitting in the waiting room, I tried to grade some student papers, thinking this might help me to relax. But the effort was in vain. After what was a rather weak effort, I put aside the assignments. What could I possibly do during such an incredibly stressful situation? Almost remorseful that I had not pursued it more forcefully during the last few hours, I stood up and began to pray, pacing across the now-empty room. After all, isn't that what ministers are supposed to do?

After a short time, I looked up at the clock and noticed that it was 11:55 AM. Being strongly impressed to relinquish Debbie—to give her up to the Lord—I started to do just that. In quite halting terms, I prayed the hardest words that I had ever prayed in my life. I told God: "I give Deb back to you. I no longer hold on to her. I want her and I need her here. But if it's your will to take her home, then do so. She is Yours; Your will be done."

As spiritual as this might sound, my follow-up request showed more clearly my fear: "However, King Hezekiah asked that you prolong his life and you did so for fifteen years. But I'm asking you for more than he received. I'm asking that you give Debbie back to me for the duration of a normal life."

I felt like this was all I could say. So I repeated the prayer again and again. Afterwards, I sensed that my burden had been released. I had prayed what I needed to, and had relinquished my hold on my wife. Looking up, I saw that it was now 12:15 PM. Just then, Debbie's bed was being wheeled out of the room. She was experiencing much discomfort and didn't tell me until the next day what had happened to her during the CAT scan.

We had been separated by a wall, keeping us perhaps thirty feet apart. The scan was given in three segments, so Debbie was also able to know what time it was. At the same moment that I stood up and began praying, she was also praying very similarly: "Lord, I want to raise my children and see my grandchildren. I don't want to die. But if it is Your will that I come home to be with You, then I want Your will to be done." What occurred next was simply incredible.

All her life, Debbie struggled with sensing God's love, as well as fearing death as a result. We linked these emotions to several very difficult circumstances in her childhood. Few people know this, but in a 1990 book on Christian doubt (*Dealing with Doubt*, Moody Press) where I included actual experiences with altered names and places, Deb gave her permission to be used as an example. She exemplified how believers could fear death, as well as question how God could really love them.

Yet, during the third and last segment of the CAT scan, marking the same time that I looked up and saw the clock, Deb said that God spoke to her. While there were no audible words, yet she never doubted that God had actually communicated with her. As she reported, He only said three words: "I love you."

But given Debbie's fear, that message was immensely important. From that moment on, she never questioned God's love, and never again feared death. She simply knew that God had communicated with her. In the almost twenty-five years that I had known her, she had never made a comparable claim of any sort. In fact, she specifically told me that it was the only time that God had ever said anything to her.

When she spoke about the incident later, I could not account for her experience in any other way except that she had been touched by the Almighty. Once while going for a walk, we were talking about this episode. I decided to give her a little test. I asked her: "Deb, on a scale of one to ten, how sure are you that I love you?"

Without hesitating, she replied: "A ten."

I continued: "On a scale of one to ten, how sure are you that God loves you?" Before she responded, I immediately thought to myself that a score of seven would indicate a tremendous change in her.

To say that her reply astonished me would be an understatement. She said: "That's also a ten."

Incredulously, I pursued my questioning. "Do you mean to tell me that, after all your past questions, you can now say with complete assurance, that you are as sure of God's love as you are of mine?"

All she said in response was a totally assured, "Yes."

I continued: "Then what does this mean?"

Again she replied rather quickly: "I'm not afraid to die."

From that day until the end of her life, she gave no indication of questioning God's love or being fearful of death. But we'll return to this subject later.

Our day at the hospital had not ended. But after another test, everyone seemed thoroughly confused. One of the doctors frankly admitted that the CAT scan had not revealed what he thought it might. Another concluded that the most likely cause of Debbie's symptoms was appendicitis.

Dave Beck had returned in the meantime. He and I questioned the last doctor for some time. We left with the understanding that further tests would be run on the samples they had obtained, and then we would receive a call with the results the next day. By this time, even if questions were all we had, they sure beat the more gruesome forecast I had received that morning! I thought I had reason to doubt the initial cancer prognosis.

Debbie and I drove home in a cautiously optimistic mood. Still, it had easily been the worst day of my life. Unfortunately, I still wouldn't know what was going on until the next afternoon. I hoped with all of my heart that the nightmare would be soon be over. But I also realized that, as bad as this day had been, it could just be a precursor to a much worse day tomorrow.

2

False Alarms

The next day, the foreboding nature of Debbie's illness continued. We were wiped out from the activities, as well as the ups and downs, that we had experienced. We felt like doing nothing but sitting together in our living room. The children were in school, and it became a time of quiet reflection.

Being of an analytical nature, I continually reviewed the possibilities. My thoughts went something like this: Deb had always had a touchy stomach. Even as a child, she was infamous among her brothers and sisters for things like holding up family vacations until she got over her periodic sicknesses. Also as a child, doctors had wanted to operate in order to remove polyps in her stomach, but the family had decided against it.

After we were married, living with her sensitive stomach was simply a way of life. Some foods were too spicy.

Others were too greasy. Large portions of any kind of food were eschewed. As a matter of fact, Deb had a little ritual at restaurants and often at home. She would almost always leave the last bite or so on her plate, teasingly saying that it was precisely that morsel that would make her uncomfortable! Then there were still the trips; almost any excursion away from home caused her discomfort of one sort or another. We traveled with medicines and peppermints in the glove compartment.

So, I reasoned that her problem was more simple than what was first thought. I concluded that the medical indecision of the day before was most likely not due to cancer, but to some form of infirmity more consistent with her lifelong ailment. Perhaps it was some sort of colitis. Or perhaps it was Crohn's Syndrome. The doctors had already told us that these diseases could cause the same symptoms. At any rate, it made more sense that everything was connected to her past.

So by the time the telephone rang that afternoon, I had pretty well convinced myself that the problem was something other than cancer. Admittedly, I also wanted fervently to believe this conclusion.

But then I recognized the voice of my wife's doctor. He did not hesitate to get right to the point. "We still think Debbie has ovarian cancer," he explained.

Still shocked, I could only repeat his diagnosis. "So she has ovarian cancer."

"No," he said patiently, "We **think** that's what she has. But we're just not positive at this point. That's why we're sending you to the university hospital for a final diagnosis."

Then he went on to explain the interesting experimental results. Having discovered strange looking cells that they thought were cancerous, other doctors had been called in to give their opinions. Before it was finished, five physicians had "voted." Three thought it was probably ovarian cancer, one said it could be that, and the last one said that he couldn't tell.

"What a strange set of circumstances," I thought to myself.

I called the university hospital to set an appointment. I even had an opportunity to speak to the chief specialist there, and again went over the options and the strange "mystery" surrounding the case. They would see Debbie in just three days.

This was a very tough time for my family. From what it seemed to us, Debbie had gone from being well to perhaps very sick in just two days! One moment I would be convinced that the doctors were mistaken. The next, I only hoped the cancer would be detected at an early stage. And it seemed that, every time the phone rang, my heart would skip a beat until we knew if there was any further news.

During this time, I called several friends in the medical profession to review my reasoning. Did any of my thinking concerning an alternative sickness make sense to them? A couple of physicians suggested that Deb had non-malignant, fibroid tumors. Then there was the doctor who favored appendicitis. But one doctor told me, "Pray it's not ovarian cancer." He went on to explain that since there are so few signs, this type is usually only caught in the later stages. The majority thought that even if it was cancer, all indications were that it was at an early stage.

With all these possibilities, we traveled to University Hospital, taking with us all the relevant scans. We sat in the waiting room for perhaps an hour, but it seemed to take all day. I tried to keep myself occupied by doing some reading. "Just a little longer," we consoled ourselves. Finally, we met with the chief specialist and his assistant. They, too, seemed just a bit puzzled by the findings.

Afterwards, they sat down and explained their conclusions. We had waited for precisely this meeting for too long. Surgery was definitely required. Apart from that, their best diagnosis was that there was a 50-50 chance of cancer. Basically the same symptoms could be produced by a host of non-malignant causes: endometriosis, Crohn's Syndrome, or some other sort of colitis. Appendicitis was now thought to be a long shot. Agreeing with some of the comments I had heard earlier, the doctors thought that, even if it was cancer, several signs pointed to it being early. All in all, the possibility that some serious, life-threatening disease might be present thankfully seemed to recede into the background.

Deb was sent to another part of the hospital for some kidney tests before we could go home. While we sat and waited, we joked lightheartedly, the relief being obvious. I hung on to her arm and hand, as if I didn't want to let her out of my sight or reach. We both looked at magazines and tried to relax.

During the tests on Debbie's kidneys, I sat adjacent to her room, pulling a chair out in the hall so I could be as close to her as was possible. I visited her between rounds. Then the attending physician was kind enough to bring me into the X-ray room each time a new set of pictures developed, patiently showing me the progress of the dye and what it revealed.

There appeared to be a congenital weakness on one side of her kidneys. But the final conclusion, after a couple of hours of testing, was that there was nothing to be worried about. After a brief bite to eat, we went back to our car and headed home. We listened to music, praised the Lord, and breathed a bit more deeply.

Now came the even tougher time of waiting for an appointment for the necessary surgery. It was scheduled for the day after Easter, exactly one week away. It would seem that we would finally be able to know the verdict one way or the other. What would the final results show? Would it appreciably change Debbie's life? How about the other five of us in the family—would our lives be changed forever? Hopefully, the whole thing would be over quickly and rather minimally. I didn't even want to think about chemotherapy. We would have to wait in order to find out. But there comes a time when you get so tired of the process that you think you are ready for what lies ahead, whatever that might be.

We tried not to involve the children in the anxiety of the moment any more than was necessary. After all, since we still didn't know what was going on, there was no reason to take a chance on upsetting anyone.

The two weeks of questioning had become a time of reflection for us. Even though the signs cautiously pointed to less than a life-threatening situation, it was serious enough for us to make the very most of our time. I went back to class for a week or so, but the professors in my department were kind enough to cover the remainder of the semester for me. In the meantime, Debbie gave up her baby-sitting.

As a result, the two of us spent virtually all of our days in each other's presence. One of the most gratifying things, I reminded myself, was that we did not have to "invent" or "force" special times during these tough moments. For years, our flexible schedules had permitted us to spend a great amount of time together. Except when Debbie was shopping or I was at the university, we spent our time together. For instance, four times a week we sat down, relaxed, and enjoyed lunch. But more than just punching the clock, we spent quality time in various pursuits. Now we practiced with a new zeal what we had been doing all of our married lives.

The pre-eminent principle in our marriage, from our dating days, was to place the Lord at the center of our lives. I have, from the beginning of our relationship, carried with me a high school picture that Debbie gave me very soon after we began dating. Still inscribed on the back are the words, "I hope we both grow spiritually and we put the Lord first in our lives."

Earlier in our marriage, we were sporadic about having devotional time together. But for the last ten years, we were quite faithful in this regard—both concerning prayer and the reading of Scripture. We had worked our way through the Bible more than once. We didn't stop now, continuing to share our faith with one another. In particular, we began to concentrate on the Psalms, mostly to encourage Debbie, since so many of her favorite passages were located there.

Over the years, this had become much more than a time of devotions. More frequently, we also used it as an opportunity to just talk to each other. It was not unusual to sit together for a half hour, an hour, or more. The children, with or without their friends, would more often than not come in during the sessions. Although we never planned it that way, we always thought it was good for them to see us spending time together around Scripture and prayer.

The next most crucial element in our marriage was to experience and express total devotion to each other. Whether privately or in front of the children and others, we left no doubts in anyone's mind that we were deeply in love. Several times a day we would hug, kiss, or express our affection for each other by the kind of things we said. Most of the time, no one else was present, but quite often someone else was there. It just made no difference because what we did was honest and in good taste.

When we sat somewhere, it was always together if at all possible, whether at the dinner table or at church. We often held hands in public, or I sat with my arm around her. We did this around the house, too. When I used our video camera, I zeroed in on Debbie and said into the microphone, "There's my girlfriend," or "Isn't she good looking?" or something similar.

We were always proud to be with each other. I really enjoyed being seen in public with Debbie. "We belong to each other" was the signal we sent to the world. We were also careful about being around members of the opposite gender, especially when we were apart. It was simply the case that no one else was allowed to intrude in any way. For our parts, we were careful not to take even the initial step towards weakening our relationship by any sort of infidelity. Our love was total, unswerving, and uncondi-tional.

It was very important to us that the children under-stand that the point of all this was not to try to impress them or anyone else. They knew that we did these things regularly and whether or not anyone else was present. For example, when they would come in during a hug, we purposely went on with it. Debbie and I believed in being honest and open about our relationship. Absolutely none of this was for show. This was simply the way we were; if anyone else cared to witness it, they could. And that was as much of a key as was anything else: we were just being ourselves—without any "show" or put-on.

Part of this was treating each other with respect, too. After all, if we didn't do so, we were sure that no one else would, either. Children are great at picking up on some weakness, and we were determined that it not be something we expressed (or didn't express!) toward each other.

As a result, we never corrected each other in front of the children. We never allowed a child to come to one of us for an answer and then go to the other parent if they didn't like what they heard, playing each against the other. We had virtually no arguments in our twenty-three years of marriage, and I don't think our children remember anything of this nature. But when something needed to be discussed, it was done politely and behind closed doors.

Once, when our oldest child, Robbie, was a teenager, he stopped by to talk briefly during our devotions (which seemed to be the most typical time the children wanted to discuss something!). Concerned that he had **never** seen us quarrel, he actually asked, "Why don't you guys argue, like everyone else?" We were quite amused that he sounded bothered by this. So we both responded with a smile, "What do you want us to do—fight?"

He responded, "Yes."

When we asked "Why?" he astounded us by saying that it was precisely our **lack** of fighting that made him think that we didn't have a normal, healthy relationship!

Following naturally from our total devotion to each other was a related principle: we talked openly about everything. No matter how private or difficult the matter, our often-repeated principle was to discuss all subjects.

We were convinced that, when two become one in marriage, a simply indispensable part of that oneness included intimate sharing. The atmosphere needed to be one that generated openness and honesty in all things.

Behind this there was the conviction that so much of what causes trouble in marriages is a seemingly small issue that "festers" just like an open wound, until it becomes seriously infected. Therefore, one key was to discuss even touchy issues before they could develop into something much worse.

We also thought that, wherever possible, even the children needed to be involved in frank discussions, both purposely being allowed to overhear our chats, as well as when we spoke directly to them. This was important not only so that we could model a healthy husband-wife relationship in front of them, but also so that they could witness the benefits of family sharing.

So these three principles framed our marriage. The priority of our relationship to the Lord, complete devotion to each other, and a total openness in our discussions were principles to which we were totally committed. Of course, this didn't mean that it was always easy to apply every single aspect of each. But we were willing to work at keeping these precepts foremost in our minds, as well as in our actions. None of this ever changed during these troubled times, either. If anything, we were even more dedicated to them.

During this waiting period, one incident, in particular, typifies these principles. Soon after it had been made clear to us that Debbie might, in fact, have cancer, she and I were alone in the kitchen. Many times I would just hold her in my arms. Sometimes I wouldn't say very much, while other times I would pour out my emotions to her. On this occasion, I felt constrained to make a brief comment. While I would just as soon not bring up the subject of death, I thought that she would want to be assured about a couple of items. It may have been the most difficult thing that I had ever said to her.

As I recall, I began rather haltingly. "Deb, I just want you to know something that I think is very important to both of us."

"What's that?" she countered.

"Well, I'm not saying that you are dying. In fact, I really doubt that you are," I began. "But, even if things are worse than we suspect, I want to make a solemn promise to you." Here I had to stop before I could proceed.

"Even if you have cancer, and especially if we are told that it is terminal, you can be absolutely assured of two things." I began to talk faster in order to end my comment as quickly as possible. "The kids will be fine; you don't have to give that a second thought. Further, I would want you to look forward to heaven."

"I know the kids will be fine," she responded.

Little did I know, but the subject of heaven had already been resolved. Deb had simply not told me yet about her experience in the CAT scan. She no longer feared death and knew that, even in the worst of earthly circumstances, she would be still with her Lord.

3

It's Terminal!

*E*arly one bright, sunny morning in April, the day after Resurrection Sunday, Debbie and I loaded our clothes and other personal items and headed to University Hospital. The drive was beautiful, with springtime growth in plain view. The dogwood and other blossoming trees were always so colorful this time of the year. The many white, pink, and red colors were not wasted on us, even if we could not give them our undivided attention.

It seemed natural to hope with everything in us that the beauty of God's nature would somehow carry over to Deb's prognosis. If only the new, seasonal life could symbolize a good medical report the next day! We talked about the Lord as we traveled along.

Over the entire trip, we specifically tried not to concentrate on the upcoming surgery. But when we did address the subject, I tried to emphasize the positive nature of the last and most authoritative medical report that we had.

"After all, didn't the chief specialist tell us that there was only a 50-50 chance that it was cancer?" I asked. Here I reviewed the data that argued for the more positive reading, a summarization that I realized I had made about one hundred times before.

"And even if it is cancer," I continued, "everyone agrees that the signs point to an early detection." I understood, of course, that I was also trying to convince myself with the diatribe, too.

Debbie didn't say much. She acknowledged my concise conclusion, but was too polite and understanding of my own struggles to remind me how many times she had already heard something similar. Who knows? Maybe she even needed to hear it herself.

In a time of skyrocketing hospital costs and insurance changes, we were required to have permission in order to arrive at the hospital one day before the operation. But that had already been arranged and Debbie was scheduled for one day of preparation and observation.

Debbie's sisters, Lynn and Judi, were to join us that first evening. They were driving down from Detroit, Michigan in order to be with us. Judi, a nurse, had taken personal time from her own hospital duties, leaving her husband with the three children who were still at home. Lynn also had to arrange her personal schedule, since she was the leader of a woman's Bible study, as well as having her husband and one child who remained at home. They would prove to be simply invaluable sources of wisdom, insight, and spiritual encouragement in the tough days ahead.

The four of us were together that first Monday night. We all sat in Debbie's room and tried as much as possible to keep the discussion light-hearted. Funny comments and family stories were the order of the evening, periodically broken by nurses coming in to perform various tasks.

The two sisters and I left about 10:00 or so. They went to their motel room and I was banished to a nearby waiting room, due to the fact that my wife had been placed in a semi-private woman's ward. For me, the remainder of the evening was spent in prayer and Scripture reading. As I recall, I tried to bargain with the Lord for Debbie's health, going to sleep in relative peace that things should be better tomorrow. I didn't even care that the couch I was on would barely have held a child and that I had to pull a chair over for my feet. I was just happy to be as close to Debbie as I was. I well knew that much of our emotional struggles are often due to facing the unknown. For good or for ill, that would no longer be the case after tomorrow.

I arose very early the next morning. It was still dark outside, but I just had to see Debbie before she was taken away to surgery. Lynn and Judi joined us a short time later. We prayed together, wished Deb well, and released her to the orderlies with a kiss.

Having been told that the surgery could take any-where from two to four hours, depending on what was discovered, the sisters and I tried valiantly to relax. At least our intentions were good. But we ended up by pacing, talking in low tones, and reviewing the medical informa-tion for the last time.

After the minimal waiting period, the chief specialist returned to the hospital room, where we had been told to wait. The three of us tried in vain to read the expression on his face before he even began to speak. But I distinctly remember his opening words, forever etched as they are in my mind.

"Well, I won't lie to you," he began, exhibiting a serious countenance. "She does have cancer. It's not ovarian cancer, though."

After a brief pause, he continued. "She has stomach cancer. We didn't remove anything, but sewed her back up. This sort of thing can only be treated by chemotherapy."

A few questions later, I knew what Judi probably already realized, due to her medical training. No, it wasn't ovarian cancer. But as bad as that might have been, my Debbie had something that was far worse. . . .

"No, there's no known cure and not much hope that chemotherapy will work," the physician continued, in answer to our questions. "I'm very sorry."

"I am, too," I thought to myself.

For the second time in less than two weeks, my world fell apart! The dreaded conclusion that we had so feared had now been delivered, and with a finality that I couldn't even begin to comprehend at that moment. After a few more questions and some medical explanations, the doctor left us to our own thoughts. With few exceptions, I remembered almost nothing he said. The grief and shock of such an announcement are simply impossible to reproduce in mere words.

At that very moment, I felt like I was in the worst possible agony. I felt like screaming. No, it was more like begging. "Please, someone, tell me I'm just dreaming. Say it's not true, after all. Tell me you mixed up the patients or that someone made another mistake. Please! I won't be angry!" But no one stepped forward to tell me otherwise; only silence ensued..

Lynn, Judi, and I sat in Deb's room, totally bewildered. Had we heard the doctor correctly? But as we exchanged notes, we found that, unfortunately, we had heard him all too clearly. If his assessment was right, Debbie was dying, and had been for some time.

In retrospect, we saw the dilemma from another angle. So that's why the first round of testing was so inconclusive. And this also explained Deb's most recent digestive problems. Perhaps most enlightening of all, that's why Deb had lost eighteen pounds in recent months, we thought from a "no-fat" diet that we had been following. The fact was that the cancer had metastasized.

Many, many tears were shed over the next few minutes. Through it all, each of us tried to console the others. The one who was most in need at any given moment received the most attention.

Once again, the questions rapidly rushed into my overloaded mind. Was Debbie **actually** going to die, then? How could it all possibly be true? Was there really no medical hope? Was a divine healing possible? Oh no! What about our four children who were all still at home? How would I tell them? I couldn't bear the thought of having to explain the situation to Robbie, Michelle, Holly, and Kevin. How could we possibly go on our normal course of life without Deb?

Still other questions came later. Would Debbie be in much pain? How long would we have to stay in the hospital? What would chemotherapy do to her? Would she even allow it? When could we see our children? How would our mothers take the news? What about the rest of the family?

One thing was absolutely certain. No matter what questions presented themselves for consideration, my mind was single-mindedly focused on a single, primary topic: Debbie's mortality. I just could not even begin to imagine a life without her presence. She was so much a part of my life. As I had told her before, we were not two people, but one. What happened to her, happened to me, too.

Right there I made what seemed to me to be a crucial mental note. Whatever else occurred, I had to be sure that I not begin to die with her. I would now have to be the chief emotional support for our children. I had no question in my mind that Deb would agree. No, that wasn't even strong enough. She would absolutely **demand** that I remain strong for both the children and myself.

This brought me back to reality. Grieve as I might, Debbie would be brought back from recovery in an hour or so. I needed to be there for her; this was not the time to mourn. Not only did I have to be strong on her behalf, but I had to make some phone calls in the meantime. In fact, they had to be made right away. I needed to be in the room when she returned and I didn't want her to hear about the situation for the first time from a phone call to a third party.

Quickly, I called my mother, who was staying at my home with our children. Like the earlier phone call to her, which now seemed so long before, she couldn't believe that the medical prognosis was about the worst possible. As I explained the situation, once again I experienced the sickening emotions that I came to associate with this sort of news.

Then we formulated a plan on how to inform the children. My mother would tell the two older ones, Robbie and Michelle. Only the fact of the cancer would be related. We knew, of course, that they were old enough to figure out what was happening and would draw their own conclusions. The question of the younger children, Holly and Kevin, was more difficult. Surprisingly, I still formulated a rational plan.

The next call went to my good friend and family physician, Richard Lane. We decided that he would pick up my two youngest children from school, take them home, and explain to them about their mother's cancer. Once again, the point would be to not provide any more information than they absolutely needed, and especially not to mention the normally terminal nature of this disease.

From a later phone call, I found out that all the children had been told at least the initial details. I was unspeakably thankful that they had all responded with a minimum amount of questions and concern, at least for now. My mother told me that Rich had simply done a beautiful job of explaining things to Holly and Kevin. And although she wouldn't say anything about herself, I also knew that she had just the right words for Robbie and Michelle, too. All of this was certainly a blessing—and one less thing about which I should be concerned.

"You don't have to worry about us here," she concluded. "You can tend to Debbie and be content that the children are doing fine." Later, my father gave me the same assurances. On the one hand, I knew that my parents were being somewhat idealistic. But at the same time, I knew that what they said was close enough to reality that I could relax just a little. They had always had a way of making blessings out of difficult situations and I was now exceptionally grateful for that quality. I could turn back to the situation at hand.

Debbie was brought into her room shortly after and I was glad that my calls had been completed. Judi, Lynn, and I had all been waiting for her, but no one knew quite what to say. The reason for this was simple: we were not sure what Deb knew and didn't want to discuss more than was necessary before she was even totally removed from the effects of the anesthesia.

By the next day, however, Debbie was acclimated once again to her room. Already knowing the nature of her disease, she then found out about its severity. Her oncologist came by for a visit. Although I had never met her before, it wasn't long before I was impressed with her, especially her empathy. She came quickly, though compassionately, to the point as she leaned over the bed.

"Honey, you have a terminal disease," she explained to my wife while holding her hand. "We cannot cure this kind of cancer. You will have it as long as you live."

Although the words stung me, too, I was more concerned about their effect on Debbie. Looking down at her, I could see that, if they had come as any surprise, she wasn't showing it.

I followed the physician out into the hallway—one of the earliest of many such discussions I had with medical personnel over the next couple of weeks. They would come to know me and my questioning nature.

"I realize that every case is different," I began. "But what is the general textbook longevity of this kind of cancer?"

"Eight months to two years," came the terse response.

The doctor explained details about related cases that she had seen, pointing out that Deb's specific variety of stomach cancer was fast-moving. The information was helpful, but again I was unprepared for yet another jolt. I was quickly realizing that I could measure my ordeal in terms of shocks—the first one coming back in Lynchburg on the initial day of testing. The second, of course, had been yesterday after the operation. Now this third bit of news numbed my mind: Deb might not be with me for very long.

Almost like an alarm had sounded in my mind at that moment, I remembered the penetrating words that Debbie had told me so long ago when we first began dating: "I've always thought that I would die young," she had said. Since then, this theme had been mentioned between us on several other occasions. Now it looked as if she might, in fact, be correct after all. Unbelievable!

Still another scare came four days later. Judi thought my children needed to be brought to the hospital to see Debbie.

"Why?" I blurted out. "Do you think she is dying right now?"

Judi only replied that, since Deb was resting calmly, it would be a good time for them to come up. But I thought I detected fear in her voice—something that she wasn't telling me. Only later did I discover that she had talked with one of the attending physicians, who had predicted that the time was shorter than we might think.

I had now been shocked a fourth time. Although Debbie was currently doing well, Judi's seeming alarm served as a rather forceful reminder that one day it might not be so. Years ago while in the pastorate, I had worked with terminally ill patients. I knew that, given the nature of these sorts of things, the next call might be the last one.

I responded by asking her how I could face my children if Debbie ever did die. Judi then shared one of the most significant insights I had heard for some time:

"Children are very resilient. They will bounce back." Her projection would prove true several months later.

The children did visit that day. Perhaps needless to say, they were very glad to see their mother. I was reminded how scared they must have been in recent days, not having seen either of us for one week, in addition to hearing the horrible news. Again I recalled how this dilemma was causing pain for many people beyond me.

On the way home from the hospital, the two younger children asked my mother and younger brother Kevin if their mom was going to die. In fact, we had been waiting for this question, and I had already "briefed" both of the adults. As unalarmingly as possible, they explained to the children that it was possible that their mother could die, but that no one ever knew that sort of thing for sure.

Once again, I was elated to hear that this answer had pacified their interests. Now they knew all they needed to about the state of the disease. Like so many other subjects, younger children often want a little information and no more. It's often we adults who insist on providing more facts than they require.

As a psychologist friend of mine, Gary Sibcy, had reminded me when he had visited the hospital during the past week, children (and sometimes adults, too) need to have threatening information "leak in gradually, rather than rush in." These words were also among the most important ones I was to hear during the entire travail, and I both repeated and practiced them often.

Over the next few days, the four of us actually had some good times together. Taking turns strolling outside among the blossoming trees, or walking Debbie around her floor in an effort to prevent the occurrence of pneumonia, we even had times of sincere levity. Once we had a private praise service in our hospital room, singing to God and praying. It is now a precious memory.

I also thought on more than one occasion about how much of a blessing Lynn and Judi had become and how much of a burden they had taken off me. The amount of encouragement, physical, emotional, and spiritual, was simply incalculable. When I had married Debbie almost twenty-three years earlier, I couldn't have asked for better sisters-in-law.

A week after Judi and Lynn came, they left for home. Judi, in particular, was required to return to her own hospital. It was a difficult parting, to say the least. As they were to tell me later, they had to face the long drive back to Detroit with the realization that they might not see their sister alive again. I was now alone in a private room with Deb, where she had been placed immediately after her surgery.

Over the next week, just like the one before it, I rarely left Debbie's side. I continued to sleep on a chair that opened into a cot, awaking regularly when nurses came in to check on her. I became a fixture around the hospital, and the nurses joked about hiring me to take care of the other patients like I was doing for Debbie! During this time, I lost fifteen pounds, mostly because I had no desire to go to the cafeteria and leave Deb alone. I ate the fruit and bagels that visitors had brought, but that was about all, periodically crossing the hall for a fresh cup of coffee. The weight loss was in addition to the eighteen pounds that I had also lost over the previous five months by following the no-fat diet with Deb, before we knew that she was ill.

Debbie slept much during these days. I would read, watch a ball game on the television, or keep a sporadic diary about what had happened, plus my thoughts and reflections on the situation. Counting various answers to prayer and blessings that we had received, as well as noting some of the lessons I had learned, also helped to keep me from getting discouraged about our situation. Sometimes I would stare out the eighth-floor window of the hospital, down on the train tracks and subdivision below us. It was warm outside and I frequently reminisced about our twenty-three years together. I thought of past vacations that occurred about this time of the year and other happy experiences together, wondering if we would ever share such moments again.

But the minute a nurse came in, my daydream was broken. I would usually hop up and assist in whatever ways I could. I wanted to understand what was being done and what I would be doing for Debbie once we got home.

The time moved on. Peace seemed to come to me more frequently during these days alone with Deb. Emotionally, I thought I was growing stronger again. To be sure, I was hurting, sometimes even severely so. But I tried to put the whole scenario into an eternal perspective. I wanted God's will for her, as tough as that might be, just as I had prayed on that first day of testing. Frequently, I thought about heaven and being able to spend eternity with Deb, no matter what else happened. Sometimes all I wished was for Debbie to be comfortable, without any pain.

Then we were given a hint that we might be able to leave the hospital in a day or so. This made us happy, but it also caused us to become impatient. We were anxious to be home again. Talking to the children and my parents over the phone got old pretty fast.

Before we could leave, however, the staff arranged a visit from a home-care nurse. I had to learn how to give Debbie both a number of medicines, as well as a liquid food supplement, through the stomach tube that had been inserted during her surgery. We went down the hall to a waiting room while Debbie slept.

During this visit, I was hit with shock number five, the last one I would get while in the hospital. The nurse was familiar with Debbie's type of cancer and gave me some additional information that I had not yet heard. I guess I had never really considered how stomach cancer killed. Now I was informed that it frequently moved either to the bones or to the lungs.

The image this invoked was almost unbearable—the first such sensation I had experienced in several days. I pictured Debbie either suffering from horribly painful bone cancer or choking as her lungs filled up. "Is this what I have to look forward to?" I asked myself, fearful that the answer was an affirmative.

Two days later we were allowed to go home. It seemed like that day would never arrive! A nurse came in with two bags filled with the initial installment of several prescription medicines and explained how and when to place each one in Deb's stomach tube. I had been practic-ing giving the food and medication in the meantime and now I had to apply what I had learned. It sounded scary, but I took notes, mostly from the sheer volume of the directions. The last thing I wanted to do was to make a mistake.

After I made a couple of trips to the car, we said good-bye to the nurses, and wrote a few notes to those who did not work that morning. Never had I seen such a highly-skilled group of medical professionals than I did at this hospital. Then I pushed Debbie to the car in a wheel-chair.

We were on our way home at last, and very excited to see our family again! Every mile brought us closer, but not without some apprehensiveness, too. How would we make it without the support of the medical team we had just left behind? Could I properly give the medicine and food that were required? When would we begin the chemotherapy treatments? And always looming prominently in my mind was the question: how long would my family have our wife and mother at our side?

4

Life at Home

We arrived home on the last day of April. How the place had changed! Besides my parents being there and "keeping house," two of my brothers' wives and my mother had totally gone through the house from top to bottom, performing a thorough spring cleaning. One of the sister-in-laws, Marla, had driven over from Cleveland, Tennessee. The other, Carolyn, lived locally in Lynchburg. Together, the three of them had cleaned the entire residence, in a grand effort to surprise Debbie.

We knew immediately that something had been done, even before entering the house. Inside, the curtains were open and the warm sun was filtering through into every room, causing a pervasive sense of cleansing light. Upstairs, the water bed had been removed from our bedroom, for fear that Debbie wouldn't be able to get up, due to her surgery. It had been exchanged for the double bed in one of the children's rooms. And these were just some of the items that we noticed. Deb was embarrassed that others had cleaned her home, but she was genuinely thankful, too.

It was obvious that much hard work had been accomplished here. Everyone had tried their best to make Debbie's homecoming as comfortable as was possible. I was grateful to see the way my family had responded to Deb—both families had already performed yeoman's service on our behalf.

But now the time for my new work had come. After carrying Deb up to bed, my next responsibility was to make sure she was as comfortable as possible, as well as beginning her tube feeding and the giving of the various medicines.

That afternoon we met our home care nurse. We set up a pole and the feeding machine, and I practiced hooking up the latter. Then I made a chart for the medicines, in order to keep track of the times that everything needed to be given. I promptly started both the liquid food, as well as the medicines. It would definitely take a while to get used to, but it all needed to be done.

Actually, I "caught on" very quickly. The next day, the feeding machine wasn't working the way it was supposed to do. When the nurse arrived, I politely explained that I thought she was setting up the plastic lines incorrectly, utilizing my meager experience from the hospital training I had received. We changed the route of the lines, and—voila!—the food flowed smoothly. Admittedly, I was very pleased.

My days began to revolve around my duties with Debbie. Food was "served" three to four times daily. After each, the bags had to be rinsed, with a major cleansing every morning. Medicines were given at least that many times, but on a different schedule. Using a large syringe, I would push the drugs into her stomach tube. Even specific amounts of water had to be given in this manner. While Deb was not eating solid foods yet, she did sip some ice water. I just had to be sure that she received neither too little nor too much liquid. **Everything** had to be measured.

All of the tasks for her were too willingly done out of love. It never occurred to me that I was performing some sort of heroic measure, as had been suggested to me by several people. I appreciated the comments, but didn't agree with the content.

Often, I would go up to our room and either sit on the bed with Debbie or kneel down beside it, usually depending on how her stomach felt at that particular moment. If she was doing okay, I would give her a hug and a kiss. But in some way, I touched her whenever I could. Besides talking about the normal sorts of things that couples discuss, I repeatedly told her every day how much I loved her and how much she meant to me.

"I love you more than anything in the world," was my most recurring statement. I don't think she minded the frequency at all, probably because she knew how heartfelt it was.

"You're the best thing that ever happened to me," was her most common response. Even though these words were repeated often, I can testify that they never lost their meaning. I treasured them every single time, without exception.

Once again I was just thankful that these sorts of words didn't originate because of Debbie's sickness. In fact, there was probably even comparatively little increase in their frequency. We had always been expressive with our emotions. Only the intensity changed.

Sandwiched between the medicines and feedings were my new responsibilities. I jokingly responded to questions about how I was doing that day with the words: "You know, I think I'm becoming a pretty good mother!" More frequently, though, I simply answered, "I'm coping." Times could be very rough.

My new duties included many of the things that Deb used to do around the house. Every morning I had a specific routine, which was difficult at first, since I was a "late night" person. I began with the early medicines. Then I got the children off to school. Holly made the lunches. Kevin let the dog out. Michelle occasionally drove the children, especially if it was raining. Then I washed Deb's feeding bags multiple times after the morning rounds, as well as cleaning the dishes. Sweeping the kitchen finished the early list.

And then there was the telephone. I never heard it ring so many times in my life! I was thankful for the outpouring of love and concern, but I couldn't always handle the large volume of calls, especially during the feedings and medicines. As much as I hated to do it, I began taking the phone off the hook during the day, often until the children returned home in the afternoon. Our family and friends were very supportive and graciously understood why I had to do it. Many of them had encouraged me to do it in the first place.

Our dinners were provided by the people in our church, Grace Evangelical Free. They had brought them to my family every night while we were in the hospital and continued to do so faithfully after we returned home. This was a huge help, since the only things I knew how to cook were eggs, pancakes, and whatever could be barbecued!

The church kept up the practice for literally months afterwards, too. Frequently, I reflected on the planning and coordination that was involved, in addition to the cooking itself. The people were so faithful! I was regularly embarrassed to witness what people were doing for us. I was reminded of the admonition of the apostle Paul: "Therefore, as we have opportunity, let us do good to all people, especially to those who belong to the family of believers" (Gal. 6:10). I was thankful.

Others occasionally brought desserts or other items. One long-time friend of ours, Eileen Holofchak, had sent home-made sweets while we were in the hospital. She also sent bottles of lotion and bathing soap to Debbie, articles that were immediately used on a daily basis. Later, she brought desserts over, but never let us know that the food was from her. When we went outside to get the morning newspaper, the kids or I sometimes found goodies anonymously left on the porch. If we hadn't recognized the design on the plates, we would never have known that Eileen had sent them.

During the day, the children were in school and Debbie frequently slept. In my time alone, my mind usually skipped from one subject to another. I reflected on one item for awhile, then moved on to the next. The strand that joined the thoughts together was a singular one: my wife was terminally ill, lying in our bed at the top of the stairway.

One detail that caught my attention concerned how those who live through the terminal illness of a loved one not only face the initial grief that comes from being a direct observer, but repeatedly face death again and again through the grief of others. So often, people would call who had just heard about the situation for the first time, or who hadn't been given the latest update. I realized that, by retelling the account, I exposed myself to some of the same suffering by reliving the episode for a second, third, or fourth time, or even more than that.

Further, hearing the pain on the other end of the line affected me by itself. I didn't want that family member or friend to hurt. Often, I was even asked why these things happen, and I would turn into the counselor! Sometimes these sorts of discussions made me feel better, and other times they added to my exhaustion.

"It's no wonder," I often told myself, "that I go to bed at night so tired and worn out!" True, I had many new duties and responsibilities, but they were not as burdensome as the emotional element that was always present.

One reaction to this multiple hurt was to take my telephone off the hook. Another was to considerably shorten the number and intensity of the details that I shared. It wasn't long before I discovered that an abbreviated account shortened my pain. But I disliked responding in these ways. Not only could someone try to call me with a serious message, but there was another related realization. Others were hurting, too. Even though their hurt was less than mine, I reminded myself yet again that the death of a beloved individual caused much pain for everyone involved.

Another reflection resulted from two seasonal celebrations. Mother's Day came shortly after we arrived home from the hospital. Debbie was doing fairly well and was able to come downstairs for a little fun. The kids and I tried to make it a special time for her. They gave her their cards and gifts while I filmed the occasion. Then I gave her a designer doll for her collection, a type that she really enjoyed. She was very happy and couldn't believe I had done that.

The second event, shortly afterwards, was my daughter Michelle's seventeenth birthday. Again Debbie was able to share in the family festivities. Cake, ice cream, and presents are always nice!

But these scenarios were a very sober time for us and it was impossible not to reflect further on their significance. Would this possibly be Deb's last Mother's Day? Father's Day would almost surely find her doing okay, but what about our twenty-third anniversary a bit later? Would she be alive for any other family birthdays? These were among the most painful thoughts I had to face during her entire sickness.

A related issue pertained to the four children. I realized with just a little reflection that I couldn't always expect them to say out loud what they were thinking. Of course they were suffering through all of this. Here and there, they provided hints as to the nature of their concerns. I needed to be sensitive to the differing forms of grief, requiring me to "read" the signs: the quiet cry in the bedroom, staying away from home whenever possible, comments about God and faith, and so on.

Many times the children wanted to talk, usually privately, on a one-to-one basis. As a result of seeking the more solitary locations for their chats, none of them probably realized how much the others were also coming to me. That was something to point out to them frequently, since it had been my experience over the years that even the assurance that one is normal is often a tremendous boost.

"That's quite normal," I regularly responded. "No, you're not 'going nuts,' honey" I would add with a smile. Usually, that was enough assurance.

On other occasions, however, I had to seek them out and request a talk whenever I thought the situation demanded it. It was on these occasions that getting a response would more likely seem like pulling teeth. It was as if, when **they** wanted to speak with me, the conversation would flow more normally. But if I was the initiator, then I would have to push a bit more.

Besides thinking about the present, I reminisced about our past, too. Vacations and other trips became a favorite topic for me. Not only did this provide some escape, but it was simply that time of the year. My classes were over and the children's would be soon. Where had we been in years past?

I recalled our yearly trips to and from Montana, where we lived for three years while I taught at a Bible college. I remembered the beauty of the mountains that started in the backyards across the street from us. I appreciated the picture postcard images of the ice-covered trees in winter, with even the small branches clad in their sparkling, frozen beauty. It was even more striking in spots where fast-moving creeks wound their ways through the trees. One summer morning when we left for vacation, it was in the middle of such an ice storm. It didn't seem quite as gorgeous then!

Debbie and I used to count the literally hundreds of deer and pronghorn (commonly called antelope) that we would see in the environs. Then there was the time I saw several elk and moose during a speaking engagement in Wyoming. Once when the family was traveling to

Washington, we watched herds of wild horses frolicking in the mountains beyond us.

Family reunions every other year on lakes in Kentucky and Tennessee were the highlight of our recent summers. Lasting a week, these were unparalleled for good fellowship and fun. The many pictures of Debbie and the children have been a constant reminder of the times we had together during those good years.

Trips to visit relatives on both sides of the family occurred at least yearly, if not more often. These took us to South Carolina, Tennessee, and back to Michigan, where both Debbie and I had been raised.

My speaking engagements provided even more excuses to get away, especially when the children were younger. A plane flight to Disneyland for the entire family was the result of a debate. Another appointment took us to a beach house on the Atlantic Ocean in South Carolina. We were also together on still other trips to Washington, Oregon, Idaho, Florida, and the mountains of western Maryland.

The highlight of all, however, was a trip to England for Debbie and me. Although as a rule, she didn't like traveling because of her stomach, she loved this vacation. The castles, cathedrals, shopping excursions, and British food caught her attention in a special way. Then I remembered that we had always hoped to go back some day. That was now quite unlikely.

It was thoughts like the last one that dragged me kicking and screaming back to reality. Deb was upstairs in bed with terminal cancer. Only a miracle would allow her to ever go on vacation again. My reverie broken, I would go back up and see how she was doing.

My normal habit when Debbie was sleeping was to check her about every fifteen minutes. Never did she call or otherwise require that I visit her. We often used a baby monitor to listen to her breathing when I was in another room. If it even sounded like she might be getting sick, I would bolt upstairs to see if she was okay. All in all, I had a tendency to stay around her so much, both in the hospital and at home, that the family gave a name to my constant practice. They began to teasingly call it "hovering." I thought of it as devotion.

Almost every day, Debbie came downstairs for a little while. The part of her regimen that she enjoyed the most was listening to "praise music" on cassette. It had started back in the hospital, with a number of people providing their favorites. Soon they were her favorites, too. Nurses would come in and, oblivious to their presence, Deb continued her quiet singing, her eyes closed, until someone nudged her!

Now it was very normal for members of the family to see her reclining in her favorite chair in the living room, music coming through her earphones, while she quietly sang praises to her God with hands upraised. The image of a mother and wife with terminal cancer still manifesting this worshipful attitude said more than words ever could! What a testimony she was to her family!

A few weeks after returning home, Debbie started eating a little solid food again, so we gradually backed off the forced feeding through the stomach tube. Then, during the next month, Debbie and I took fairly regular walks down the street and back again. I was hopeful that she was regaining a little of her strength. Regardless, the walks were necessary to keep her from developing pneumonia.

It was often during these strolls in the warm outdoors that we discussed some of the spiritual aspects of Deb's sickness. On one occasion, she recalled her experience during the CAT scan, reaffirming her continued assurance of God's unconditional love for her. She never again wavered on this subject.

Talking about the same experience while on another walk just a few days later, she explained to me that the knowledge of God's love totally convinced her that she had no condemnation before Him, all based on the finished work of Jesus Christ. As a result, she pointed out once again that, for the first time in her life, she did not fear death.

Deb had been receiving weekly chemotherapy treatments and was responding to them. She had also been eating three regular, although undersized, meals per day. As a result, we had totally discontinued the forced feeding. One day in mid-June, the doctor surprised her by asking if she wanted him to take the tube out of her stomach! I don't think much could have made Debbie any happier. No return to the forced feeding! Only pills instead of the syringe!

"What do you think?" she asked me, barely able to contain her enthusiasm.

"It's your decision," I countered. "I wouldn't want you to have it inserted again some day, but you do whatever you want."

It didn't take her long to respond. "I want it out," she said to the doctor.

She closed her eyes and it was gone in just seconds. Deb opened her eyes and asked: "Is it out yet?" She couldn't believe that there was only a little mark where the tube had been.

"That will heal in a few days," declared her physician.

For days afterwards, Deb's elation continued to be obvious. She now began to regularly go outside and sit on the back porch. She even looked healthier.

Not only did the doctor take her feeding tube out. He also gave her permission to go to see my brother Keith, his wife Marla, and their family in Tennessee. We could stay for a one-week vacation. I had said that it would take a miracle for her to ever travel again, and this was exactly what I wanted to hear. I was excited, as well.

Four days later we left, along with our two youngest children. Debbie even drove a fair amount of the distance. We had a simply wonderful time. We relaxed around the house, often resting on the back porch and sharing meals together. Keith, Kevin, and I fished a few times, and were lucky enough to land several large bass, as well as some big catfish. (But who would believe us about this subject, anyway?) Even nine-year-old Kevin caught a large bass. Marla, Debbie, Holly, and cousins Sarah, Tracey, and Missy shopped, making some good "catches" of their own! The kids also got to swim and visit with their cousins.

Most of the time, Debbie could be found up and around the house. Throughout the week, she ate regular meals, though with a growing amount of painful indigestion.

We returned home on a Saturday evening. The next day, Debbie was not able to eat. Little did we know, but this signalled the beginning of the end. Keith later told me that, when we left, he told Marla that he did not expect to see Debbie alive again.

5

Of Vitamins, Miracle Cures, and Humor

Sooner or later, victims of cancer are usually approached by well-meaning friends, acquaintances, and loved ones who want them to try some remedy that is often portrayed as being more likely to heal than conventional medical methods. Very frequently there is a pattern here, and the slogans are repeated by many, sometimes countless times over.

"Traditional treatments don't simply fail, they actually speed the dying process along. In particular, chemotherapy kills; it just ruins the immune system."

"Don't even ask your doctor about this. Just start doing it. Of course medical doctors will disapprove. They are simply not trained in these areas and can't abandon their medical training or their livelihood."

"No, these methods are not medically approved. But what the doctors are proposing doesn't work anyway. So what's the difference? You may as well try it."

Along with the claim that these non-traditional methods work better than the standard ones come some simply
incredible reports on behalf of the treatment being
proposed. Two sorts of claims seem to predominate: miracle cures to begin at home and trips to exotic lands in
order to try new remedies. Once again, the testimonies
tend to sound quite similar.

"I know this man who had incurable cancer; in fact
his doctors told him there was nothing else he could do.
So he began such-and-such and in his next check-up, just
three months later, all the cancer was gone. The doctors
were dumbfounded and said they couldn't explain what
happened. Here's what he did . . . ."

"I know a place you can go. A friend of mine went and
they cured him of his cancer. Granted, the remedies are a
little wild, but they work. Here's the phone number . . . ."

As the informant sometimes admits, the treatments
are often "wild" and perhaps even counter-intuitive.
Coffee enemas? Drink aloe-vera water? What kind of tea?
Powdered what? Only this particular brand name of product? Three eight ounce glasses of this per day? Special pills
that I can only get from you? Anti-oxidants can cure cancer
when nothing else works?

At least three categories of remedies should be identi-
fied here, as suggested in the title of this chapter. I think
that by far the most commonly recommended claim
concerns the use of large (sometimes massive) amounts of
various vitamins, usually A, C, and E. But these are by no
means the only ones that are encouraged. Others explain
that laughter is an outstanding therapy that has been
proven to heal. Still others suggest certain (sometimes
rather exotic) operations or other miracle cures. During

Debbie's sickness, I received piles of books, tapes, articles, reports, and product samples.

Now I do not want to be misunderstood here. I am not criticizing these people or even their ideas. Some of them really do seem to have documented results from accredited physicians and other well-trained health care professionals. I read several such medical articles and reports that were very impressive. I even took some of them to my friends who are medical doctors and argued on their behalf. It is true that some remedies are simply better than others and a few do have experimental confirmation of one sort or another.

It is also true that we are in the comparatively early stages with some of these remedies and some changes may indeed be forthcoming in the medical community. For example, a number of medical doctors have changed their views in recent years concerning the use of certain vitamins, and some even prescribe them for their patients.

Another factor was in operation here, too. The vast majority of those who called us were well-meaning friends and loved ones who only wanted the best for Debbie. Their sincerity was unmistakable. I would never denigrate their response, or the hurt in their own lives over our situation. Very few tried to make a profit or otherwise gain from our situation.

But problem areas also need to be recognized. A couple of factors, in particular, make these sorts of proposed remedies very painful for the terminally ill patient and their families.

For one thing, the claims made on behalf of the vitamins frequently conflict. For example, different reports variously praise and condemn chemotherapy. Some encourage vitamins along with lower levels of chemo. Others declare that any of the latter can speed the loved one's death. The suggested dosage differs widely, as do the claims made on behalf of the healing effect of vitamins. Many insinuate that healing will take place if certain steps are followed, while others simply say, "it can't hurt." Unfortunately, the affected family has more decisions to make than they can perhaps handle, given everything else that is happening.

"Miraculous cures" also conflict with each another, since one must choose between options. When a trip is required, one has to think about the children, as well as other family members. Is it justifiable to spend much of one's remaining time away from home, all for the briefest glimmer of hope? What should be said on behalf of the sick individual's comfort?

Further, all of these "super remedies" can cause a fair amount of guilt, too. Have I done enough for my loved one? Is it possible that if I just read one more article, or talked to one more researcher, that we might find a cure? The tendency is always to think that everything is one's personal responsibility—"It all depends on me!" Choosing the best treatment, the proper dosage, how much one should rely on traditional methods, whose advice should be followed and whose should be rejected, are all decisions with consequences. In fact, it is often claimed that **only** a certain, specific remedy will work. But then here's the other problem: nothing short of healing is allowed. An added problem is that, when one's loved one has only a short time to live, one wishes to concentrate on the person, not on dosages, mixtures, and concoctions.

At any rate, I think ours was a fairly typical case. Shortly after arriving home from the hospital, we received telephone calls and visits from numerous sources, the largest number being those who encouraged me to give Debbie various sorts and dosages of vitamins. I took a crash course on the subject. After doing a fair amount of study, and talking with a number of professionals of various sorts, I did decide to pursue the possible benefits that might come from this avenue. I purchased some liquid vitamins and, after checking specific dosages with a physician, I began placing them in Debbie's feeding tube on a daily basis. I also started giving her fairly large doses of vitamins C, E, and acidophilus.

Then we graduated to a new level. A good friend went out of her way to help educate us concerning some of the benefits of vitamins. She delivered piles of relevant information. Then she brought her own juicer, along with some of her own "stock" to our home, and showed us how to use it. She left the machine there for weeks, periodically checking in with me as she made her "rounds." All of this was without charge. In particular, I made carrot juice for Debbie. Surprisingly sweet, especially when chilled, Debbie didn't mind drinking it when she could. I also gave Debbie glasses of aloe vera water.

Then we began to hear about other possibilities. I called a medical doctor in Virginia who had reportedly traded traditional methods for vitamin treatments, giving patients enormous amounts of vitamin C. A friend told us about another doctor at one of the top medical schools in the country who had also "switched" to vitamin treatments. Articles told about still more doctors, with traditional medical degrees, who had done the same. Some of them provided details of controlled testing.

Checking out these reports the best I could, I just couldn't tell whether they really achieved the results that were reported. Sometimes it was incredibly difficult to even get details.

"Who referred you?" I was asked once. "We must be very careful not to give out information to just anyone because some authorities want to close our operation." I have to admit, that answer didn't give me a lot of satisfaction!

At least a portion of the "vitamin trail" seemed to be a largely unsubstantiated journey for us. There were too many unverified reports and wild tales that were simply false. On the other hand, I concluded that certain vitamins could really help us to remain healthy. But then again, Debbie was not healthy. Neither traditional nor non-traditional methods seemed to be working to her benefit.

Others suggested that the human body has the ability to heal itself and that humor is one of the chief means of unlocking this potential. Considering this claim, and having done some reading on it in the past, I figured that at least it wouldn't hurt to apply it. Even if it wasn't able to heal, laughter would still be good for us. In fact, it had always been a part of our family's relationship—so why not now, in spite of the seriousness of the situation?

For several nights before we went to the hospital for Debbie's surgery, we watched tapes of the Three Stooges, specifically in order to help reduce the tension. Although Deb had never been particularly fond of this sort of humor, she saw the value of it and enjoyed my hard laughing, even if she was not inclined to participate directly. For my part, I appreciated seeing her smile no matter what the reason, especially when she broke into an all-out giggle. Few things were as rewarding.

Even after the diagnosis, we seldom missed a chance to be funny. I encouraged Debbie to participate, too. There were many occasions when it was appropriate and when it unquestionably helped us to relax. In fact, Deb often initiated the laugh.

While setting up the IV pole in our bedroom, Deb couldn't help to take a good-natured poke at the rising medical costs in our society. Glancing up to see me move the pole closer to the bed, she remarked with a wry smile: "That thing probably cost us $200.00. I'll go out in the woods and get a stick."

Once when I started to leave the room after attending her for a while, she said: "For a minute there I thought I was losing my room service."

Debbie was not even above making herself the brunt of the joke, even in rather sad circumstances. Seeing how much weight she had lost, she looked down at herself one day and remarked: "Well, will you look at the thighs on that girl." Another time she referred to herself as "Queen for a day."

One day we looked out of the window and watched our nine-year-old son, Kevin. Trying to fill a small swimming pool with the hose, he moved the nozzle to the other side. When we later asked him about the move, he explained that he did it in order to level the water! Even Debbie got a good laugh out of that episode.

One of the times when Deb's younger brother Fred came down from Detroit to see her, the two of them enjoyed a great many laughs by recalling several of their childhood pranks. First one would tell the story, followed by the other: the time they skipped school and got caught at home by Mom; pretending to be sick in the bathroom so they wouldn't have to go to school; throwing an entire pile of newspapers under a tree instead of delivering them to their customers.

Deb also teased with her older sister Judi about the times they slept in their double bed and Deb wanted to wrap her feet around Judi's ankles. Judi didn't appreciate it and had wished there was a board in between them. Strangely now that Deb was sick, Judi again slept with her for just one night. During that evening, Deb again turned over and wrapped her legs around her sister!

Rather late in her sickness, I brought her home after a trip to the doctor's office and carried her up to bed. As family members came in to see how she was feeling, she kept us laughing for some time, primarily by teasing twenty-one year old Robbie. But to this day, we can't remember her comments and, unlike the other occasions, I didn't write them down. I often wished that I had done so.

We always appreciated the teasing and laughing, right up until the end. Although we could hardly claim that we considered it to be useful in the healing process, it was something that we needed. It was just so good to see Debbie laugh. And without question, we needed it, too.

Neither did the "miracle cure" route contribute much to our search for a healing. Once I called to check on another nontraditional therapy in Mexico that had attracted many Americans. I was told that it had helped several people with stomach cancer, at least one of whom had been totally healed. Once I got the information I needed, I was also skeptical. Besides, Debbie said that she had absolutely no intention of going!

We inquired about other well-known cancer treatment facilities around the U.S. And of course, I called the American Cancer Society. But in each case, we were told that nothing significant could be done in Debbie's specific case.

I did acquire much of the more traditional literature on cancer during this time, too. Doing some reading, I was surprised at what I found concerning stomach cancer. Debbie had none of the signs associated with this variety. In fact, she was virtually the opposite of every characteristic! "One more mystery to store away," I concluded.

Another friend of ours whose family member had been treated successfully for lung cancer at a major cancer center in New York offered their home to us.

"Come and stay with us and we'll drive you downtown for the treatments. Bring the entire family and stay as long as you need to, at our expense," they told us. Especially knowing these people, we were tempted to take them up on their offer.

Then one of our chief physicians called and told me that Debbie had been cleared to go to the National Cancer Institute in Maryland. They could try certain experimental drugs that were not available anywhere else. But once again, we were clearly informed that there was virtually no hope of healing Debbie.

One night during our walk, I spoke to Debbie about the last two options. We considered them carefully. But Deb did not want to go away again, and for more than one reason.

"I just got home from two weeks in a hospital," she sighed. "I simply can't make myself travel long distances with almost no hope of healing. Besides, what about the children? I don't want to be separated from them again."

She saved her last salvo: "Besides, if the Lord wants to heal me, He can do it here. He doesn't need help from any cancer centers."

What faith, I mused! The last time I heard her answer like this, she was in the hospital. A psychologist had visited her, to see if she wanted to learn any pain control techniques.

"I'm not really in much pain," she responded. "But even so, I'm trusting God to heal me, but only if it is His will."

As we walked quietly out in the hall, I asked the psychologist what he thought. He turned to me and remarked just briefly: "Her faith is very strong. She'll die with it." I didn't know whether to be upset with his pronouncement, or be proud of Deb's faith. I chose the latter, since I had heard the former enough times by then.

So, in spite of all of our research and testing, we settled for the traditional route. We decided to try chemotherapy, but Debbie rejected the harsher versions that would cause nausea, vomiting, and hair loss. After our consultation, I spoke alone to the oncologist. I was told that the combination we selected would very possibly keep the cancer in check for a while and make Deb a bit more comfortable, but that there was no chance that it would defeat the cancer. Again, Deb was undaunted.

"If God wants to heal me, He will," she affirmed. "But if not, the chemo won't do it, either."

More than once, she also repeated a similar statement: "If any healing occurs, it is of God and not due to vitamins, medicine, or doctors. God can use any or all of these, but He's the Source of any cure."

During the weeks to come, Debbie was given a total of six chemo treatments, from which, thankfully, she had few ill effects. During that time, we met probably the most professional group of nurses I've ever known. Their combination of skill and friendliness made the atmosphere there as nice as it could possibly be.

Interspersed around the chemotherapy treatments, we also had to take a few trips to the hospital across the street. Once, the stitch that held Debbie's stomach tube broke, threatening to cause the line to come out entirely. It was a scary time, since all we could envision was a return for further surgery. On another occasion, the tube plugged, keeping the medicine from entering.

Once we stopped in the hospital gift store. While Debbie was looking around at several little novelties, I reflected on her love of shopping. I had often teased her about out-walking those who had gone with her over the years, always in search of a bargain for the children or me. She was more "in her element" in a mall than any other place. Her idea of a good time was to wander around several stores, watching for sales and comparing deals. I noticed that even her sickness didn't affect these desires!

In the middle of June, we visited the oncologist's office once again for our regular appointment. I cautiously anticipated the monthly report on Debbie's blood work, that also included her cancer count. It is very difficult for me to explain since I am not given to these sorts of convictions, but in preparation for this particular visit, I thought that the Lord had given me the knowledge that Debbie's cancer count would be cut in half—from over 1100 (as per her last visit) down to 600. I specifically envisioned the second number.

But when we spoke to the doctor before the chemotherapy treatment scheduled for that day, he informed us that the report from the laboratory hadn't arrived. I was a bit crestfallen. Were my musings, then, really from the Lord, or only private affairs?

It was later that same day that Debbie's stomach tube was removed. The doctor came back to see us while Deb was hooked up for her therapy. "By the way," he informed us, "I did find the blood report after all. Debbie's cancer count has fallen from 1166 to 636." Admittedly, I was shocked!

I then asked: "Is it merely a **good** sign, or is it a **great** one that the cancer count dropped almost 50%?"

The doctor got a strange look on his face that I couldn't quite decipher. Shaking his head affirmatively, he acknowledged that it was very impressive. But I distinctly remember wondering why he seemed to be less than excited. I'm not sure that I wanted to know why he didn't seem to share our glee. Perhaps there were reasons that kept him from being equally impressed. At the time, if that were the case, I really don't think I wanted to know. I was too happy in our new developments. And I knew that Debbie was elated. We praised the Lord several times, both in the room and on the way home, and meant every word of it.

Perhaps needless to say, I could hardly believe what I had just heard about the cancer count. I had not said anything to Deb about my previous thoughts, because I didn't want to give her any false sense of hope that could be dashed by the next report. But now I wanted to tell her of my experiences. She was interested in the account of her lower cancer rate, as well. It was difficult for us to deny that, for whatever reason, the Lord had allowed me to know that He was still in control.

I remember that for days after that experience, I was hoping that the Lord would reveal some even greater victory. But that same sense never returned. I even did what I almost never did and asked the Lord some time later for a sign that Debbie would get better. Oh, how desperately I wanted to receive it! But the sign I asked for never materialized.

The trip home from the doctor's office that day was a real blessing for both of us. What were probably the two most positive events in Deb's sickness had occurred. Her much-hated tube had been taken out of her stomach, and we learned that her cancer count had gone down drastically.

Before we arrived at home, Debbie told me that she had learned four great lessons so far. When I asked what they were, she enumerated them for me: (1) God's love for her was unconditional; she was justified in His sight. (2) Accordingly, she still had no fear of death. (3) More than ever before in her life, and mostly through her singing, she was learning that praise to God was exceptionally important. (4) God was awesome!

I simply marvelled at her testimony—and her faith.

Through all of this time, Debbie was more than a warrior. She was absolutely stoic, and even funny. She had always been cooperative, through tube and medicine feedings, as well as when I stuffed her with vitamins. Now, on top of everything else, she was the source of edifying blessings given to others, revealing the grace that God often gives to His dying children.

6

Family and Friends

During Debbie's illness, to say that my family received an outpouring of care would be a misnomer. We were simply inundated by visits, calls, cards, letters, and prayers. The expressions of love were just phenomenal. I'm sure that I didn't even begin to comprehend the attention we received, especially behind the scenes.

We received so much mail that it now occupies two piles in a good-sized box. The most common comment I heard was that prayer was going up to heaven on our behalf. Literally dozens of individuals and churches promised prayer. At one point I counted people from twenty-some different states and seven foreign countries among this number. And this is just those that I knew about and could recall some time later.

Many of the details were humbling. One church in Florida called for a twenty-four hour period of fasting and prayer. A church in Michigan gave our requests very special attention. Prayer chains in states such as Arkansas and Virginia were passing on requests concerning Debbie. An entire class of children at a local elementary school sent Debbie home-made get-well cards.

A pastor in Michigan, Doug Hornok, called me one day and promised: "My family is making a covenant with yours. Not a day will go by as long as Debbie is sick that we will not pray for you."

A former colleague called very early in our ordeal and said "since I've heard the news today, not one minute has gone by that I have not prayed for you. I mean this literally. I will not be one who promises prayer but doesn't do it."

To know that so many Christians were so serious about our struggles was a tremendous lift to me, especially hearing their voices, seeing their faces, and knowing how much they meant what they said. The offers to help in every imaginable way were likewise sincere.

The literature on death and dying agrees that one should almost never tell someone going through the situation, "I know what you're going through." Especially after the loss of a spouse or a child, the griever doesn't want to hear: "I know exactly what you mean. Years ago I lost my grandmother and . . . ."

This is surely not to say that all deaths are not painful—only that some are generally more so than others. The griever often wants to cry out, "No, you **don't** know what I'm experiencing. Come back and talk to me when you have." Of course, it is the pain and emotion crying out here, not disregard or judgment of others.

But even if the friend **has** lost a spouse or child, you still want to point out, "Yes, but you're obviously over it, I'm not." I often felt these sensations.

However, I did experience an exception to this general rule. Often I gravitated to those whom I thought had or were suffering similar amounts of hurt. I felt an "emotional comradery" towards these persons. I learned from them and experienced their pain, as I think they did mine. Several conversations fell into this category.

One call was from someone I didn't even know, but whose wife was in the final stages of cancer. He simply wanted to share with me some things he had learned, especially regarding help that was available to cancer patients. Not having crossed this pathway before, I appreciated his advice and personal experience.

A good friend from Talbot School of Theology, Doug Geivett, had been co-editing a book with me when Debbie got sick. During the past year, even before my family's experience, Doug's wife Diane had been fighting a cancer bout of her own. "It's pretty strange," the two of us mused more than once, "that we are editing a book on the subject of miracles and, in the process, both of our young wives have been struck down in this manner!"

Two other colleagues, Donald Cudworth of Liberty University and John Feinberg of Trinity International University, were suffering intensely while their wives struggled with Huntington's Disease, an exceptionally debilitating and terminal sickness. Don visited me very early and loaned me a book that had been tremendously helpful to him. I was not the only one to make use of it over the next few months. John and I talked on the phone rather regularly that summer, both telling the other how the books we wanted to write about our wives might possibly be more influential than any others that we had ever written. Interestingly enough, John was another of the contributors to the miracles volume!

Then there was the family at church, Kip and Cindy Hughes, whose son Adam had been close to death several times in the previous two years. Not only did they sympathize with my plight, but they even had to visit the same hospital we were in for tests of their own, precisely while Debbie and I were staying there. Later I met Adam for the first time, and the four-year-old stunned me by his testimony.

"I pray for your wife three times a day," he said.

"He really does," confirmed his mother. "I don't think he has missed yet."

My son Kevin had been praying for Adam during this same time, too. After hearing Adam's comment about Debbie, Kevin's prayers for Adam became even more meaningful. To this day, Kevin still prays for Adam every day.

My children's friends came for visits, too. No one could believe what was happening to our family. Robbie's closest friend, Michael, still visited the house about as much as he did before, when he was known as my "other son." Kara, Rob's girlfriend, was really affected, primarily because she had spent so much time talking with Debbie over the previous year or so. Michelle's boyfriend, Bryan ("spelled with a 'y,'" he always reminded us), had just begun to get to know our family.

So it was that we had the support of so many friends around us. Further, our relatives also came to our aid in just an incredible way. Debbie and I both had large families and each of the other brothers and sisters visited us during the summer, sometimes more than once. Not only did they spend some wonderful time with Deb, but they helped around the house—cooking, cleaning, washing clothes, repairing, and building. A number of projects were started and completed. My lack of home improvement prowess had always been a joking matter of mammoth proportions in my family. My outdated and meager collection of tools was the brunt of many a joke.

"Go borrow tools from Gary, he has plenty."

"Kevin [my brother] uses tools, Gary uses books."

Perhaps needless to say, I was more than thankful for all of the assistance!

The most convicting thing in all the visiting was the sacrificial aspect. Several family members took time off work to visit and help us. The week that Lynn and Judi spent with Debbie and me in the hospital has already been mentioned. They were to contribute far more at a later time. The house cleaning that my mother, Marla, and Carolyn had accomplished has also been mentioned. My brother, Kevin, did several projects around the house. He, too, would figure even more heavily in the future.

My parents took care of the children during our two week hospital stay and I never had to worry about a thing with them around. Answering the telephone alone was almost a full-time job at our house! My father and Kevin provided taxi service several times and over many miles. Deb's brothers Dave, Fred, and our brother-in-law Don worked on several projects around the house. Although we were always close to each of these families before Deb got sick, we unfortunately never realized the degree of our commitment to one another until these difficult times were upon us.

As difficult as these months were, I really tried not to neglect our children, even though it was definitely not "business as usual." We continued to try to eat our meals together, work schedules permitting. We also fit in some games and movies on what we called "family nights." Once, when a family member stayed with Debbie, I took the kids to play miniature golf. On the Fourth of July, we enjoyed some fireworks together at a neighbor's house.

Other relatives also helped to give especially the younger children a lot of attention. Time out for ice cream, a special lunch with an aunt, dinner with grandparents, other meals out, swimming in the community pool, staying overnight with friends, matinee movies, many shopping safaris, books to read, walks, and a shoulder to cry on were all a normal part of their life. A particularly difficult load was hopefully being lightened just a little.

During these times with family and friends, I learned a number of important lessons. I realized that we often take our loved ones for granted. A hot meal when no one in the house knows how to cook is something we really began to look forward to, and our church provided dinners for several months. My mother and sister-in-law Carolyn also brought a number of dinners. To see what others were willing to do for us, as I've said, was a humbling experience.

I also realized that we shouldn't wait until a family death to get together with one another. Even the kind of compliments and warm statements that we repeatedly heard during these months should not be invoked by terminal illness. I realized that I was always willing to compliment a friend or family member to a third party, but seldom did I directly tell the person I was complimenting.

One of the most important lessons to impress me during this entire episode in my family's history was the sanctity of life. To me, life had always been sacred, a gift from the hand of the Creator. This applied to the small things in life, too. I had always cherished a bird's song, the scurrying of a squirrel among the leaves, the sun, or the spring blossoms on a dogwood tree. But now I added other items to that list: a warm meal, a good night's sleep, a game, a card, phone call, or visit from a friend, a relaxed look on Debbie's face or the squeeze of her hand in mine. Being surrounded by loved ones in a crisis also brings contentment. As my mother wrote in a diary she kept during these days, "It feels so good to be surrounded by family during a crisis."

Another thing I learned was that burdens are not meant to be shouldered alone. Others are both strong and trustworthy; one should learn to rely on them. It was during these troubled days that this point came through "loud and clear," especially since I was simply unable to do everything that had to be done. Little by little, however, I realized that others could be trusted to do things that Debbie and I had always done ourselves—particularly concerning the children. As one item after another worked out, I began to realize that I could give some control to other adults who also loved my family.

As I think back about everything that happened, one of the areas that pleased me the most was the large number of beautiful compliments that Debbie received during these days. Many of them were mentioned on the telephone, while others were written in cards and letters, both to Deb and to me. I passed on to her as many of them as I could. Unfortunately, she never saw some because they were reflections that arrived after her death.

One relative told both of us that ours was the best marriage they had ever known. One of my in-laws sent a card and said to me, "Thanks for being such a good husband to Deb." That comment was very meaningful during her sickness, since I frequently found myself second-guessing various matters.

For years, Debbie had worked while staying at home, by baby-sitting. Now we just began to realize how much of a lasting effect she had had on the families of those whom she served in this manner. One of the mothers had physical symptoms that were similar to Deb's, but it had turned out to be noncancerous. She was devastated by the opposite results of Debbie's testing. Another family credited Debbie with being so helpful with their baby who was later discovered to be autistic. Though not known at the time, we were told that Deb's advice in some trying circumstances was just what this young couple needed.

We were also contacted by several of my ice hockey players whom we had gotten to know so well while I coached for nine years at Liberty University. They had known both Debbie and me because of our open-door policy. One couple actually said that, when they got in a fight, they literally stopped and asked themselves, "What would Gary and Debbie do?" To say that this greatly surprised me would be an understatement! Later another person told me almost the same thing. One player wrote and said, "Debbie was without a doubt a very giving lady to share her family with a bunch like us. We are grateful for her example, and may we show the same love with those God brings our way."

We received other sorts of comments, too. Some shared their hurt with us. One very close individual wrote to us in eloquent terms, quite early in Debbie's sickness:

> I am "in the valley" this morning. I feel defeated and sad.
> I try to read Scripture and it doesn't penetrate into my

mind to comfort as I would desire. I know from past experiences, this is a temporary "lull"—the peace of God continues to remain . . . . Fear pierces my heart. We look for some glimmer of hope, some confirmation that things are not as critical as they seem. But the messages we continue to receive only confirm the darkness of the hour. I know I must run to the promises You have given us, Lord, and cling to them in sheer faith, despite not understanding . . . . [T]here are times when my soul screams "Why, Lord?" How can this work out for good? . . . We know You are leading us all *very gently* through this trial—but at times, the flesh rebels in pain. I know, too, I won't be feeling this way in a few hours—Praise the Lord—it comes, overwhelms, and it passes! Calm and peace are restored.

Coming as it did from one of the most spiritually-mature believers I knew, I was heartened by this writing. Besides its obvious honesty, I rejoiced in its wisdom. Knowing this person well, it was really true that dark times such as these were, thankfully, short-lived. The person looked not to the present, but to the time "down the road," perhaps only a few hours away, when the mood would pass and God's truth would again take over. But so often, we wallow in our emotions without the long-term look of those who know that their God is indeed trustworthy.

Time and again, throughout this entire ordeal, I would remind myself of this truth. It's simply a fact that we do not always know why things happen as they do. But for those who cling to our great God, we know that He is trustworthy even when we don't understand.

Days, weeks, and months later, I also received other testimonies about the effect that Debbie had in the lives of those she touched. Perhaps the most moving was from a young lady who had become a friend of the family, and who credited Deb with helping her over some potentially serious emotional struggles:

> I wasn't afforded an opportunity to say "goodbye" or to tell her how much she means to to me and how I do love her. All at once my mind is flooded with memories of Debbie. . . . This was the beginning of the end of my depression and doubt. . . . For Debbie to share her family with me the way she did so often was worth far more than the over-priced advice of many counselors. . . . I loved dining with you. The family devotions were great (new to me). I would sit and talk to Debbie as she prepared the evening meal. . . . God alone knows how truly grateful I am for the times I had to share with Debbie. I am thankful for the way my life was blessed because of her. I look forward to seeing her again. I pray that the God of all comfort will keep you in his care.

"Wow!" I thought as I read this letter. I was reminded how easy it is to underestimate the effect that we can have on people's lives. How often we're bothered by what seem to be interruptions when people seek our help. Yet, testimonies like this one show how we need to be sensitive to opportunities that cross our paths. With the Apostle Paul, we need to "not become weary in doing good . . ." (Gal. 6:9). As the letter said, only in eternity will we know how we have ministered in the lives of others. And as Paul finished his same verse, "for at the proper time we will reap a harvest if we do not give up." Knowing Debbie, she probably never would have had any idea that she had done so much in this particular situation.

Other kinds of influence were also manifest in Debbie's life. A relative wrote the following words:

> I could not help but reflect on several ways in which Debbie influenced me in my roles as wife and mother.

. . . Debbie was always an example to me of flexibility. She was willing to accommodate herself to the needs of her family . . . . She was also flexible in her ability to overlook the faults of others, and was an example to me of someone who could 'live peaceably with all men.' Debbie was a good mother. . . . That thoughtful attitude toward her children made an impression on me and helped shape my attitude toward my girls. . . . One more way in which Debbie influenced me was in her home-making skills. . . . These are just a few very practical ways Debbie influenced me. When December 8 {her birthday} arrives I will remember them, and her.

Probably the subject that cheered me the most during this time was the prospect of seeing Debbie again in eternity. This idea was captured in a number of cards and letters to us. One card from friends depicted a beautiful heavenly scene on the front. The inside left quoted Psalm 32:7, while the verse on the right side read as follows:

> May you be comforted in your sorrow,
>   Knowing that eternal life,
>   Is in the Kingdom of God.
> And while a loved one has now parted,
>   You will always cherish memories
>   Of your time together
> Until you, too, enter the Gates of Heaven,
> Where you'll share your love forever.
>   (Lawson Falle Limited, Canada)

Receiving this card was the highlight of that day. I took it out often to read it again.

Terry Miethe, a long-time friend and colleague wrote the following:

Debbie, your precious wife and mother, is much better off directly in the Lord's hands than in the hands of us mortals. She has settled her destiny. Our loss, which is great indeed, is her even greater gain! We *must* see her passing through her eyes in Glory! We must go on living to see that she did not live life in vain—*assuring that she did not* by seeing that *we live ours for God*! . . . Never forget, we are all so much richer because of her life!

It was this heavenly theme that buoyed me so often and would become the single most comforting theme in my thoughts about Debbie. It was nice to be reminded of it so often by my family and friends. I knew that Debbie was living in eternity, walking the very halls of heaven. I also knew that she had already seen the Savior who had died for her and who had given her the assurance that she received in the CAT scan. I also realized that she was now living in His light.

7

One Week to Go

The week at my brother's house in Tennessee had been a very refreshing time for my family, with relative normality. Debbie had gone shopping almost every day and the children had a great time swimming, fishing, and visiting with their cousins. We needed the break.

The morning after our return, the family attended our home church. It was the first time for Debbie since her operation. We were conscious of the fact that we wanted to praise the Lord for Debbie's good health during the previous week. But Deb said as we were preparing to leave, "Let's not stay too long after the service. I don't want to attract attention or be asked to talk about what has happened." We agreed to leave during the closing prayer and told the children to be ready.

As the service came to an end, I let Debbie set the pace. Strangely enough, she did not leave on cue. Instead, she lingered just long enough that some friends came over to talk. Soon the crowd swelled. I stepped away a bit with a few men, while Debbie talked to the women. Glancing over to her repeatedly, I could see that she was speaking openly, apparently relaxed. She confirmed this later.

Although I couldn't hear details of what she was saying, snippets of the conversation told me that Debbie was talking about the awesomeness of God, and adding her testimony to that fact. I never found out exactly what was said that day, but whatever it was, it was powerful. Two of the women, both of whom had been suffering through some serious troubles of their own, later related to me that this ten-minute conversation had transformed their lives.

When I expressed surprise that such a brief talk could have such an effect, one of them added: "I mean my comment quite literally. It has forever changed me." The other confirmed the same with an affirmative nod of her head. I was astonished, but excited.

Just over a week later, on the Fourth of July, Debbie was dehydrating. She begged with me not to take her to the hospital. The next day, I took her to the doctor's office and she received two liters of water and nutrients. She had not been eating since our return, and in her weakened and dehydrated condition, I had to carry her from our bedroom to the car and back again.

Early in Debbie's sickness, it had occurred to me that one way to measure what was happening to her was to enumerate the several shocks that we had experienced— events or reports that shook me to our very being. In every instance, the news had been given to me privately, without Deb being present. During this trip to the doctor's, I experienced the sixth such shock. After the doctor saw her, he took me out in the hall.

"Debbie doesn't look very good," he began with a grave expression. "I don't think she has very long to live."

The news forced its way into my mind like an explosion. "But I thought that the medical prognosis called for eight months to two years," I questioned. "How long does she have, in your view?"

"Perhaps one to two months," he responded. He gave me other details to which I listened, but they were really superfluous compared to what I had just heard. "I'm really sorry," he concluded.

The next day I brought Debbie back for more water and nutrients. Again the doctor asked me to step out into the hall. And again I began to feel anxious.

"We got the results of her blood work. The cancer is in her liver," he began. "And I can tell she's a bit jaundiced. I'll have to downgrade yesterday's diagnosis in light of this information."

"How long do you think she has now?" I asked.

"I'd say she has one to two weeks," he said with a saddened countenance. The oncologist had always shown the utmost empathy throughout our plight.

Shock number seven hit me! "Only one or two weeks before my Debbie leaves me?" I asked myself. "Is it really possible?"

Later that morning I asked him another question, since I knew Debbie's family would be interested. "Her two sisters are coming for a visit in two days," I informed him. "They plan to stay for about a week, but they aren't exactly sure when they are leaving."

"Well, it could be over by then," he added.

Immediately I made some phone calls while Debbie's treatment was being completed, just as I had the previous day. Then, while Debbie remained asleep, I went down the hall and tried to encourage a young mother who had liver cancer. Debbie and I went back home and I carried her up to her bed.

After laying her down and making sure she was comfortable, I kneeled down beside her bed. "I love you more than anything else in this world," I said, thinking about how much time the doctor had told me she had left.

But Deb corrected me: "No, you didn't say that right."

Not knowing what she meant, I asked: "What do you mean?"

With closed eyes, she pointed up to heaven and responded: "You need to love God first, then me."

Once again, I marvelled at Debbie's faith. Here she was, dying, and she still exhibited so clearly her trust in her Lord!

During the last visit, the doctor had suggested putting Debbie back in the hospital. "For one thing, she will need to get one liter of water every day." I looked over at Deb for her response.

"Please, no. I don't want to go back," was all she said.

"I'd like to keep her home," I responded. "Her sister Judi is a nurse and she can give her the water."

"If you can do it, you're welcome to try," he said. "In fact, it may even be better that way. It's just not the way most people do it."

In retrospect, I made the right decision to keep Debbie at home during this entire ordeal. For more than one reason, I was glad I did so, too. It was her wish to return to her own bed in order to be with her family, and I wanted her to be as comfortable as possible. Further, I think the family members obtained benefits, as well. For one thing, the children would not have been able to see her as frequently in the hospital. I am convinced that the more natural death is, the easier it is to deal with its consequences, both in one's own life and with loved ones.

From the time Debbie's sisters Judi and Lynn arrived (along with Judi's children Noelle, Megan, and Ryan), I felt relieved. Although I didn't say much about it, I had felt much of the burden for Deb's medicines, feeding, baths, and especially the trying emotional times when she didn't feel well or when we talked. The latter were true blessings, but they produced a certain amount of pain, too.

The sisters immediately began to get us more organized around the house, as well as sharing in the responsibilities with Debbie. While both of them spent much time in the bedroom, Judi chiefly took it upon herself to take care of the baths and the intravenous water feedings, as well as some of the medicines. Lynn also helped with the baths, while taking over around the house. She did the cooking and washed most of the clothes. We teasingly called her "Sergeant Lynn." In fact, as much as possible, we tried to inject humor into our daily lives.

Noelle added immensely to the atmosphere around the house. Having jettisoned her plans to take a summer school class in her college curriculum, her good-natured teasing made life appear as much like normal as was possible. She played games with the children, took them shopping, and watched many a "kiddie-movie." All of this contributed to keeping a fairly regular environment around the house. Everything she did came with a huge smile. For once in my life, I had to admit that going shopping even helped the situation! As one of Debbie's shopping partners, Noelle had learned her craft well! Her many gifts for the kids were an added blessing.

These were significant months for the children and Noelle did as much as anyone in cultivating the surroundings at home. Talking to Michelle and Holly, in particular, was exceptionally important. They had always been close and she had a way of calming many troubled situations. I had so many things to think about at that time, and I deeply appreciated the burden that she took off of my mind. I knew that the children were in good hands.

One subject that continued to come up in my mind was that I had never let Debbie know how much time she had, according to the medical prognosis. It was the only subject that she considered to be "off limits" and she had made me promise long before never to tell her. I still thought she should know, and several experienced people, including Judi, agreed that I should tell her.

So I had a dilemma. My desire was to let her know, but I respected her express wish not to be told. I knew what I would say myself in the same situation and I also knew what I had said about the topic on other occasions, but she didn't agree. My mind was made up to place her wishes above mine. Further, her doctor advised me not to tell her, in light of her own request. I never did.

At the same time, I'm quite sure that Deb knew what was happening. While in the hospital she told me that she thought "terminal" meant that she had ten to fifteen years to live, while telling me not to correct her. But once she got home, the situation changed. She began to instruct me concerning which children should receive which of her possessions. She wanted our two daughters, Michelle and Holly, to get her dolls. Then she suggested that I give our two sons, Robbie and Kevin, some of her jewelry, or something else. She wanted me to get her wedding rings.

Once, very late in her sickness, Judi discovered her out of bed and standing by her dresser, taking off her wedding rings and placing them in her jewelry box.

"Why are you doing that?" Judi inquired.

"Because I don't want them to take my rings by accident when they come to get me," Debbie answered. "Gary will forget to take them off me," she finished. Few comments broke my heart like Deb's matter-of-fact response.

So we concluded that Debbie must have known that the time of her death was imminent. Otherwise, her comment about taking off her rings didn't make much sense. Besides, I reminded myself, the literature often agrees that the dying person knows of their impending death, even when that information is withheld from them. So all of these indications from her would just be normal.

During this time, Debbie had been eating almost nothing. This was not by choice, but her tumor had grown so much that it now affected her digestive system to the point that she could not digest her food even when she did eat a few tidbits. We realized that she was basically starving. At first one of the doctors gave us the impression that, in her weakened condition, she might not last past twenty-five or thirty days without food. But Debbie proved us all wrong.

Although it was an incredibly tough decision to make, we thought that we should be wise and plan for what would be, apart from a miracle, Deb's inevitable death. I turned the preparations over to my brother Kevin and sister-in-law Judi. While Kevin visited area funeral homes, Judi made other required decisions. I had very little part in the whole thing, which was what I desired. I often remarked what an incredibly difficult burden they had removed from my shoulders, and at the expense of pain on their part, as well. The two of them did a simply excellent job. Of course, Debbie knew nothing about any of this.

A high point in an otherwise tough summer came one night in July when the worship team from our church came by to give us a mini-concert. Debbie and I had only been in church twice since the diagnosis the previous April and she missed the worship portion of our service, which she enjoyed immensely. Desiring to be a blessing to her in any way they could, they brought the singers and instruments to our house for an old-fashioned "singspiration." We pushed the family room furniture back against the wall and joined in the praise.

That evening was indeed a fantastic blessing to those of us who participated. Song after song ascended in praise to God. Deb's favorite was one of the numbers that the team performed. As they finished, the leader, Scott Baker, asked if they could do anything else before they left. Debbie requested that they sing her favorite number a second time.

As the music began, we were all moved beyond expression by what we saw. With eyes closed, Debbie tried to raise her arms, but could not do so. Sitting next to her, I reached over and lifted them for her, holding them aloft during the entire song. I doubt if there was a dry eye in the entire room. For months later, the worship team referred to this selection as "Debbie's song."

When the members were leaving, I stood in the doorway in order to thank them. But I was shocked as they passed, thanking us for the blessing that **they** had received! Then one of guitarists told me that one of his sons had died at the age of ten years, and that his birthday would have come in just a few days! Again, I felt a comradery, as well as empathy for the man's pain.

I had been watching Debbie, as well as myself, during the preceding weeks and months. I had a theoretical interest in the famous five stages of death and dying, as popularized by Elisabeth Kübler-Ross in her ground-breaking book by that title (Macmillan Publishing Company, 1969). She theorized that terminal patients often progress through these phases: denial and isolation, anger, bargaining, depression, and acceptance. What is not as well known is that Kübler-Ross did not think these stages were written in stone. They could co-exist, occur out of order, or not at all.

In thinking over my experience so far, I reached several conclusions. Debbie and I had both experienced denial, especially over that initial, two-week period before the operation, but not much longer than that. Neither Debbie nor I had experienced much, if any, anger. On the other hand, we both tried to bargain with God, at least a little bit, as with my "Hezekiah prayer." Neither of us was depressed.

I think Debbie's chief reaction to the knowledge of her terminal condition was emotional isolation. She would talk if someone said something to her, but it was usually fairly brief. And the amount of her normal discussion also lessened. That was how she most frequently dealt with the pain associated with the prospect of leaving her family, as well as her physical discomfort. I'm sure that both sorts of suffering contributed to the fewer words.

Quite quickly, we both came to accept what was happening as God's will, too. This process (or stage) happened relatively early for us. Neither of us thought it was something to blame God with. Neither did we need to know why this was all happening to us. I often mused on the fact that this response was very strange for me, since I always asked questions and tried to figure things out. This time, however, my thoughts hardly ventured in that direction, even a little.

The various family members took many opportunities per day to go in and speak to Debbie, often sitting with her for long periods of time. The older children, who had somewhat avoided these situations earlier in the sickness due to the pain involved, now went in to see her more regularly. On several occasions, Robbie sat with her alone and talked. I continued my "hovering," as Lynn and Judi called it.

For her part, Debbie regularly responded to the added attention. Once she lay with her head in my mother's lap, an occasion the latter would not forget. Often she watched movies with the other women. Sometimes she reminisced about humorous times in the past. But usually she slept. The longer the sickness lasted, the longer this was the case—often for twenty to twenty-two hours a day. Lynn, Judi, Noelle, and I would take shifts sitting by her bedside for long periods of time.

Debbie suffered very little physical pain and took very little medicine for it. I was unspeakably thankful for this, to say the least, especially given what could have been the case. She often dealt with her discomfort by taking hot baths or by placing a heating pad on her back.

Towards the end, Debbie made it a point to tell me a number of times how she felt. One morning, she rolled over slowly, put her arm around me, and told me that she loved me. A few days later, she said, "I love you more than anyone in the world. And I'd marry you all over again—either here or in heaven."

These words were incredibly meaningful to me, and I wrote them down after she said them, even as I had recorded many other items over the previous few months.

Just a very few days before her death, I asked Debbie a question that was important to me. She had always been a superb mother, but not once in her entire sickness had she shown any signs of emotional pain at the prospect of leaving her family. For example, she didn't call the children into the bedroom and give them any instructions, or have some sort of tearful parting. I often wondered whether this was due to her isolation response, or if it was the calm that she experienced when the Lord communicated with her during the CAT scan. So I decided just to ask her.

"Are you suffering any emotional pain?" I questioned.

"What do you mean?" she asked.

"Given your sickness, are you suffering with regard to me, the children, or other family members?"

She was brief and to the point. "No," she responded.

"Is there anything at all that you want to say? Anything?" I persisted.

"I love you," she said.

The words were extraordinarily meaningful, coming so late in Deb's sickness. But I insisted on getting an answer to my earlier question. "What else?" I asked.

"That's all," she concluded.

Although I still think that Debbie used emotional isolation as a means of shielding herself from some of the pain, I also concluded that she suffered remarkably little emotional distress. This fact, especially in light of the committed mother that she had always been, was nothing short of remarkable. I credited this development to the Lord and His revelation to Debbie that first day of her ordeal, just as I am sure that she would have done. She accepted her death and all its ramifications. Given her previous fear, that is something she could never have done before that experience.

A day later, Debbie fainted. Judi and I both grabbed her so she didn't fall, and we discovered that her body had become very rigid. "She's gone, Gary," shouted Judi. Given Judi's hospital experience, this scared me. But before I really had much time to think about it, Debbie revived. We weren't sure what had happened. It occurred again the next day.

We knew Debbie's death couldn't be too far away. Given her previous condition, she had gone far beyond the medical estimates without eating. Thankfully, she didn't report being hungry.

But now we had another problem. Judi's leave time from work was used up. She had been at my house for almost five weeks and her hospital wanted her to return. However, she wanted to remain until the end, for Deb's sake. Who would give her the intravenous water and nutrients that she took every day?

"When the Lord answers my prayers, He usually waits until the very last minute," she told me. "So Debbie will probably remain alive until the very last night I'm here."

Two nights later it was Judi's very last night. She had stayed as long as she possibly could. She and her daughter Noelle were leaving for Detroit in the morning. They had gone downstairs to watch a movie. It was about midnight and I was lying on the floor next to Debbie. Although I was just beginning to doze, I was awakened by Deb's loud sighing. Since it sounded rather abnormal, I went downstairs and called Judi. She came up immediately and got her stethoscope.

A minute later Judi looked at me and pronounced, "Deb's not breathing. Talk to her." We both grabbed a hand and started talking to her a bit frantically. Noelle was talking, too.

I returned to my favorite theme that Deb had heard so many times over the last four months. "I love you, Debbie," I repeated over and over again, "more than anything in the world."

Checking her heartbeat again, Judi announced, "Now she's breathing again." We both continued our refrains. "You're going into the arms of Jesus, Deb," called Judi.

"I love you more than anything in the world," I added.

Several times over the next few minutes, Debbie stopped breathing, only to begin again a moment later. Finally, after about fifteen minutes, she stopped breathing for good. "She's dead," pronounced her sister.

Then Judi told me something that I will never forget as long as I live. Listening through her stethoscope, she could hear what we could not. "Whenever she stopped breathing," she began, "and you told her that you loved her, she started breathing again. That happened more than once. She was fighting it."

Deb had expressed her love for me to the very end!

8

Forever Loved

*A*lmost seven weeks after we returned from our one-week vacation in Tennessee, my beloved Debbie passed away. The day she died, August 9, was her forty-fifth day without food. It was also about a month after our twenty-third wedding anniversary.

She had died early in the morning and those of us at the house finally got to bed about three hours later. Judi and Noelle were now able to stay for the funeral about three hours later. Again it was Judi and my brother Kevin who made all the final arrangements and decisions. I felt inexpressibly thankful that I didn't have to get involved in these matters.

That same morning I felt like some physical labor would be good for me, to keep my mind off of having to go to the funeral home that afternoon in order to make sure that all was in order. So I began cutting the lawn and actually felt good doing it. My neighbor, Mark, came over and, wanting badly to do something for us, insisted that he be able to finish the job. I let him do it.

I absolutely dreaded walking into the funeral home that afternoon. But I still was not prepared for seeing Debbie. Over the next couple of hours, I had to walk out of the room many times in order to regain my composure. Later, my children arrived and that was also exceptionally painful for all of us. Just seeing their heartbreak hurt me severely. But I gave each one of them their space and let them grieve the way they chose, keeping a watchful eye on them. After all, that would be my job in the future. Other family members helped and once again took much of the burden off of me.

By the next night, virtually all of the brothers and sisters from both sides of the family had arrived in town. Before it was over, all eleven appeared. In addition, literally hundreds of friends and other family members came to visit, which was more than we had expected, especially in the summer when most of my colleagues and students were away for the season.

Before the funeral service began the next day, I went up to the open casket for the last time, something I had done perhaps dozens of times over the last two days. Leaning on the side, I mumbled some words to Debbie. Unfortunately, only I could hear them, at least with human ears. "I love you with all my heart," I said to her, also for the last time. "Good-bye for now, until I join you for eternity in heaven." Tears blurred my vision as I walked away. A handkerchief was my constant companion.

Jerry Falwell and our pastor, Mark Fesmire, performed the funeral service. It was a beautiful tribute to a godly woman who loved her Lord. I had decided long before that I wanted to speak. I realized it would be incredibly difficult, but I knew that Debbie would want me to share her testimony of the last four months of her life. I also thought that few times would afford such an opportunity to minister like this one.

When we reached that part of the service, I walked up to the podium, handkerchief in hand. It was probably the most difficult thing I had ever done in my life, especially with the casket right in front of me. There were two incidents, in particular, that I wanted to report. I told the crowd about Debbie's time in the CAT scan when she was totally convinced that the Lord had spoken to her. I related how she no longer feared death after that experience. I also explained about the day when I brought her home from the doctor's office after being told that she had about a week to live. I explained how, when I said that I loved her, Deb told me that I had to love the Lord most of all. From watching the faces of those present, I knew that her edifying testimony had made a powerful impression.

Afterwards, Dr. Falwell delivered the message along with an outstanding eulogy. In part, he said:

> Yet, I don't know of any family in which I have witnessed more of the grace of God at work and more of commitment to the will of God among the family than the Habermas family. Actually, there are two families involved here and they are all very close. They have in the past four months closed ranks, they have joined hands and hearts together. And so, I suppose likewise I don't know a family in which there is more support. Gary and the children had a crowd there—many coming hundreds of miles at times to stand by, to pray, to minister, to encourage. And then Gary . . . . in this last 120 days, his family, his neighborhood, his circle of friends, have come to know him as a devoted husband who did **everything** a human being can do in an hour like this one. I thought his words

here a moment ago were the best possible sermon or eulogy that could be given for Debbie.

I appreciated the comforting words and I know the rest of the family did, too. Indeed, it had all been a Herculean emotional effort.

That night, fifty family members came over to our home. We had shared a meal that afternoon, and now we sat down and watched a comedy together. Everyone thought that we needed a break. But that night all but my brother Ron and his family left. What a contrast! My children and I were almost alone. The biggest change was that, sick or not, Debbie was not there. And we missed her so much!

The next day, Ron's family left for Arkansas and we went back to Keith and Marla's home in Tennessee for a visit. We had about one and a half weeks before I had to return for the beginning of school, and we wanted to relax a bit.

We had a great time. We swam, fished, enjoyed some sporting events, and visited. My son Kevin not only caught his first bass, but it was a big one, weighing between three and four pounds. (And this is no "fish story!") I most frequently retreated to the back porch that Debbie had enjoyed earlier in the summer, and read books. I also caught some nice bass of my own. It was just what I needed before going back to the grind.

While we were in Tennessee, we had an experience that reminded me that, just because Debbie's death had just happened, this did not mean that we were therefore exempt from other kinds of bad news. My oldest son, Robbie, who had stayed back in Virginia, called one night to tell us that there was a terrible storm in Lynchburg. In fact, as we were to find out later, two persons even died in it. In the process, our house got flooded. A number of my books were ruined; carpets were soaked. We returned to a wet home that needed some additional work.

In later reflections, I have pondered this phenomenon that often seems to occur. As graphically portrayed by the flood, sometimes "when it rains, it pours." Over the next several months, we were forced to deal with a number of items besides our own emotions. Some of these were huge, while others were only nagging.

For starters, immediately after our return from Tennessee, and in the midst of the flood remains, our washing machine broke down for the second time that summer. (Earlier it had stopped working the very same week that Deb and I were in the hospital for surgery.) No sooner did we fix it than another part broke—the third time something had happened to it in four months! Now it needed a major repair. This was followed by our hot water heater "going out" on us, as well as a toilet that required fixing.

Much more seriously, we also had two more family funerals over the next several months. This was rather strange since we had had only one other funeral like this in our twenty-three years of marriage. Debbie's mother, Joyce Wrobel, died first. She had been sick with many different ailments over the past twenty years, including cancer, a few heart attacks, congestive heart failure, sugar diabetes, very high blood pressure, and kidney failure, the latter requiring dialysis! She was even in the hospital with the kidney and heart problems while Deb was sick. I went to Detroit with my two oldest children, Robbie and Michelle, for the funeral, marveling at the Lord's goodness in allowing Joyce to live so long with all of these problems.

Just two months later, my grandmother Mildred Jarvis (affectionately nicknamed "Nin" by the family) also passed away. I had lived with her and my grandfather "Geep" while I was attending college and they had always been second parents to me. Debbie and I had stayed with them throughout our marriage in our annual trips to Detroit. It was a tough few days for us even though Nin was 89 years old, and had lived a full and wonderful life. Having been sick for the past two years, this was not a shock. Again I returned to Detroit, this time conducting the funeral with the help of my brothers, three of whom are ministers, and her pastor.

In the middle of these problems, we had more sickness in our family than we had for several years. While nothing was serious, we constantly had to deal with the fear of many that they were also terminally ill, a common problem in situations like ours.

Interestingly enough, I think all of these tough circumstances that came about after Debbie's death made us stronger rather than weaker. We faced them all with God's help, one at a time, and I don't remember anyone asking the "Why us?" questions.

While working around issues like these, we tried to let our life return to as much normalcy as was possible. Meals were still being brought three days a week by church members, while I tried (usually in vain) to make up the difference on the other nights. Two women who cleaned houses for a living, Kathy Germeroth and Martha Shuppe, insisted over my protestations to periodically let them clean our house. "We're not saying it's messy," they explained, "everyone just needs help sometimes." I felt better when I remembered that they really hadn't ever seen the inside of my house, so it wasn't (as far as they knew) because they knew it was messy!

We still received numerous cards, letters, phone calls, and other encouraging contacts from people, especially during holidays and birthdays, the normally tough times after a family member dies. I treated these contacts with mixed feelings. On the one hand, it was heartening to witness the outpouring of attention and concern. However, receiving these notes also caused pain, as one relived certain episodes or feelings in life.

It seemed to me that the most pain occurred when these reminiscences came suddenly, without preparation. When I was ready for a discussion about Debbie, there was much less risk than when I stumbled suddenly upon some remembrance. As a result, I was tempted to respond either by controlling the conversation so that nothing unexpected arose, or by avoiding the situation altogether, in fear that further suffering would result. But then, I felt guilty for not appreciating what was being done for me by people who cared. Such was but one example of my world of mixed emotions after Deb's death.

Certain events that unexpectedly reminded me of Debbie also stung. Once, late in the summer, our family went to an amusement park as another chance at a "get-away" for the children. Two friends who accompanied us, Gary and Lori Sibcy, were walking ahead of me. Without warning (as if they needed to say something to me first!), Gary put his hand around his wife's waist. All of a sudden, my emotions rushed in, since that was always the way Debbie and I had behaved in public. It was a difficult moment.

One interesting question around our house was between those family members who wanted to see pictures of Debbie and those who didn't. I was one of the ones who favored it, leading me on an expedition to search through family photo albums and unsorted piles of pictures, on a hunt for the "perfect" photograph. In this way, I collected quite a number of memorable snapshots.

I thought I was also ready for our collections of "Family Films," the name we gave to our eight years of motion pictures, usually taken during vacations, birthdays, holidays, and other important times. Since I was usually the one who took the pictures, I often zeroed in on Debbie and made comments about her: "Look at that pretty woman," or "There's my girlfriend" or something similar. But twice I stumbled by accident on these moving pictures and the emotions were almost overwhelming. "She's actually alive and moving," I said to those around me. To this day, I've not watched them again.

In many of these pictures, I was surprised by the number of times that I was holding Debbie's hand, or had my arm around her. I probably never would have recognized this except for the recent teasing about my "hanging around" her when she was sick. "I was always hovering!" I realized with a smile. At our first Christmas without Debbie, my daughter Michelle took a number of the photographs that I had culled and put them in a little album for me. I enjoyed it often.

The children and I learned a number of things about ourselves those initial months as we went through life together. Sorrows and happiness, talking through things together or being alone, we experienced all of it. Stress and joy alike took several forms.

Grief from missing their mother was probably the most common reaction that I noticed. I often discussed this and other similar subjects with them, both singly and with more than one child at once. On one occasion after I had put Kevin in bed for the night, I walked by his room and heard him crying. I found him lying on his stomach, his chin on his pillow, staring at a picture of Debbie that he was holding in his hand! Tears rolled down his little cheeks as he sobbed quietly.

"What's wrong?" I asked, as parents often do, even when the problem seems obvious.

"I miss Mommie," was all he said. After a little talk, he put the picture down and went to sleep.

All of us had dreams about Debbie, often very regularly. I remember once having several in a single night. Unfortunately, Deb was always sick or just about to get sick. The dreamer usually had the sense of trying to warn her, and worried about having to watch her die a second time. Even so, it was also nice to "see" her alive. But the next morning, there was also some added grief.

Frustration and even a little anger were also obvious on occasion. Interestingly, the child would usually not direct the feelings at anyone or anything in particular, but it seemed to be more of a "floating anxiety" that manifested itself first here and then there. Then it dissipated on its own.

As a family, we continued to get a great amount of enjoyment from our Sunday morning church service, and the worship portion, in particular. We simply relished the praise songs, and we were all able to sing thankfully to God without regret or malice. It had always been Debbie's favorite segment and it continued to be ours, as well. Most of all, the melodies that spoke about God's awesomeness were the most comforting. Holly frequently got water in her eyes, and they were truly tears of joy. Without exception, I sighed whenever the praise portion ended. Occasionally, I was warned ahead of time by a member of the music team that they had chosen "Debbie's song" for that week.

A close relative of grief—loneliness—was my constant companion, especially during the early months after Deb's death. I'm sure this was the case with the children, too. I very often reflected on the fact that I could well have had the best children, family members, and friends in the world. They contacted me often—calls, cards, and other forms of communication. Everyone wanted to know how I was doing, and that was gratifying. Yet, when the phone stopped ringing, after the mail arrived, and when the house was dark, I still went upstairs to an empty bedroom. This was the chief sensation that I noticed. The conclusion was plain and simple—I just missed Debbie tremendously much. During this time, I often said to my mother: "I wish I could have just five minutes with her, alone."

For the first three or four days after the funeral, I had no clear sense of Debbie's presence, perhaps because of my confusion and the depth of my grief. But immediately after that, I had the strangest sensation that she was with me wherever I was. It first began at my brother's house in Tennessee and then continued after we arrived home in Virginia. I sensed this the most when I was alone in our bedroom, usually late at night. I'm willing to grant that this was some internal desire or wish on my part, just a feeling. But all I can say is that it frequently felt quite real—just like Deb was, indeed, "looking in" on me.

Although I didn't discuss the subject much with the children, I was not the only one who had the sensation that Deb was still with us in some sense. The week after the funeral, Robbie was home alone. His friend, Mike, came over to visit him. While they were talking, the subject of Debbie came up.

"Why can't loved ones just do something to show you that they're still around and that everything is all right?" Rob asked. "Like, why can't they knock something over?"

"I don't know," Mike responded. The discussion ended.

The next day, another friend, Rick, was over for a visit. Rob had told no one about the previous day's conversation with Mike. While he and Rick were sitting in the kitchen, without moving around, the heavy salt shaker suddenly fell off the top of the stove with a bang. It startled the two boys.

"Ah . . ., do things like this always happen around your house?" Rick asked, obviously puzzled. To our knowledge, this had never happened before.

One of our nieces, Mary Beth, had not been able to attend the funeral because she was recovering from the effects of a car accident. She had always felt guilty that she had not come anyway. Months later, she told us that she had also dreamed about Debbie, but that it seemed like much more than a dream. Deb "came" to her and told her that she was doing fine and that Beth shouldn't feel guilty about not coming. It had been a great relief to her.

We tried very hard to keep Debbie in our daily conversations. I even went out of my way to do this on a regular basis. We never denied the facts in any sense, but spoke openly about her sickness and death, and encouraged the children to do the same. I wanted things to appear as natural as possible around the house. There were no issues to avoid. I also wanted to let the children down more easily instead of there being a huge gap in their experience. I certainly didn't want them to think that talk about mom was somehow "off limits."

So not only did we discuss the situation of the past summer, but we would also joke about Debbie, since laughter had always been such a large part of our lives. Sometimes my daughters Michelle and Holly would want to do something that they didn't know if I would allow, like cut their hair. Playfully and without warning, I would often say something such as: "You know your mother wouldn't want you to do that." Or I might look up to the ceiling and say, "Did you hear that, Deb?" Everyone would laugh.

Overall, I was exceptionally thankful that the family's response was as "calm and collected" as it was. Even with the reactions that we experienced, and the things we had to work through, it seemed that the pain was easier to bear after the funeral than before. Without question, the uncertainty was lessened afterwards, due to the nature of Debbie's illness. Friends who knew us well all thought that, since Deb had spent almost the entire time at home, we had done much of our grieving even before her death. As a colleague and former counselor told me: "I've never seen a family respond so well or so quickly to such a difficult situation."

"Well, we've had hundreds of prayers on our behalf," I responded. "God has answered them and spared us a lot of grief." Indeed, God had sustained us throughout, especially during the worst moments. We didn't know why Deb died, but we knew that God did know. And that made all the difference.

9

Job and Me

Many times throughout Debbie's sickness, while she was lying upstairs on our bed, I thought about the case of Job, the Old Testament believer who wrestled with such a severe dose of suffering. This was a recurring meditation in my life. It was definitely **not** that I thought I had suffered as much as he did. It was just that I had often written and lectured on this famous man whose name is almost synonymous with pain, and, frankly, I wanted to know if the lessons he learned could in any way be applied to my situation.

In other words, even though I hadn't suffered as much as had Job, was what he learned practical enough to help me, thousands of years later? Or to say it still another way, I had said many times that Job's lessons **really worked** in real life predicaments. Now I had a chance to actually prove it! Could I "put my money where my mouth was" during what was easily the toughest time in my entire life?

I started by remembering a few of Job's problems. Maybe this would make me more appreciative of the remedy that he discovered. There was no question that Job suffered greatly, both physically and emotionally. On top of all this, he couldn't understand why God did nothing to help him. Why was God so silent? Couldn't God just reach down and heal him any time He wanted to? He was the God and Creator of the universe, wasn't He? But now the situation had lasted far too long. It didn't seem like the suffering would ever end. Yet, we are also told that Job's trials taught him fantastic truths that completely transformed his life.

Checking the Book of Job once again, I reviewed his situation. Although he was a righteous man, Job was tested by Satan with numerous calamities. One major problem was not enough! His domestic animals were either killed or stolen by outlaws. There goes the family livelihood! Then his servants were murdered, too. Then the evil touched his own family. All of his children were killed in a desert storm (Job 1:13-19).

Then phase two of the suffering kicked in, and the pain moved closer to home. Satan tormented Job with personal sickness in the form of painful sores from his head to his feet. Either from the itching or from the oozing of the sores, he had to scrape himself with a piece of broken pottery. "Curse God and die," his own wife counseled him (2:7-9). In spite of all of this, Job refused to sin by charging God with the fault of these multiple tragedies (1:20-22; 2:10).

Job didn't have the luxury of sitting in a classroom and philosophizing about his dilemma in some theoretical, detached manner. Neither did I. He was forced to live through his struggles and pain. So was I. But I didn't suffer as much as he did. Since he personally "paid the price" that he did, his experience should be quite instructive for me. As I said, I gravitated towards the advice and comradery of others who had lost either spouse or children. So, could Job's conclusion be applied to my own situation with Debbie? I wanted to know how well it would actually work.

After awhile, Job began to challenge God. Several times he demanded his right to have a hearing before the God of the universe. He even requested a debate on the subject (Job 13:3; 13:21-22; 27:2). Job's major question was quite a normal one: "Why am I suffering the way I am? What could possibly justify this horror?"

God responded in chapters 38-41. He spoke to Job and challenged him to answer an entire host of questions— sort of like a final exam. More than once, God asked Job if he could solve the problem of pain and suffering (38:13-15; 40:7-14). Understandably, Job didn't have an answer.

It is instructive that God never answers Job's main question, a typical one that we all ask from time to time. He doesn't tell Job why everything has happened to him. I think this tells us something very crucial and that it is even one of the keys to the entire issue. If God had provided a philosophical justification of suffering, could Job even have understood it? We're not talking about graduate school here, but an audience with Almighty God! But perhaps a layman's answer would still not have been understood by Job, or perhaps worse, wouldn't have done what Job most wanted or needed.

After all, don't the textbooks say that we shouldn't

rationalize with those who have just lost a loved one? Although I sometimes enjoyed philosophical discussions with my friends during Deb's sickness, usually I wanted no part of this sort of banter. I had no time or patience for it. After all, this was not just a theoretical situation! I wasn't interested in the three leading theories on the subject. I was hurting! If I knew this, wouldn't God? Maybe God knew that such an answer, on whatever level, was exactly what Job **didn't** need!

Whatever the reason why God never gave Job an answer to his main question, one thing is crystal clear. In the end, Job was entirely satisfied. But why did he abandon his protest against God? What had he learned?

Job came to understand that God could do anything, including giving an explanation for the suffering in the world. First, Job realized that God was omnipotent—he confessed that God was all-powerful (Job 42:1-2). Indeed, only God could perform all the things that He had just asked Job to do, including solving the puzzle of pain. Next, Job realized that the problem was actually with him—he simply did not understand the areas he was questioning (42:3). This realization must have hurt his pride! But he was honest enough to admit that he had lost the debate. After his "showdown" with the Lord, Job declared that all he could do was repent. He now despised the position that he had previously taken (42:6).

This wasn't just some mental conclusion on Job's part, either. It cost him something. He had been humbled. He had to relinquish his previous objection. Even more, he needed to act further on his decision and repent. All of this, he did willingly. What in the world could he have learned to make him do these things? What changed his mind so drastically?

We can now summarize what Job learned in his encounter with the Lord—that which became the foundation for his liberation and peace. **Based on what he knew about God, Job now realized that he could trust God even in those things that he still did not know.** In other words, Job concluded that he already knew enough about God to realize that there was a good reason(s) for his suffering, even if he did not understand what it was. He could trust the One who **did** know why it all had happened.

Therefore, Job was satisfied without ever knowing why God hadn't answered the question about his suffering. And we must remember that he made his decision even while he was still afflicted, before God blessed him (42:10-17). So it wasn't all the forthcoming blessings that made Job repent; his change occurred first.

I had realized long before Debbie got sick that there was a tremendous principle here for me to learn, as well. The times when I knew the reason why pain and evil occurred, it was so much the better. I realized that Scripture provided many of these reasons, for which I was thankful.

But even when I **could not** figure it all out, or when God seemed to me to be so silent, I also knew that I still had to trust Him. Why? Because I knew more about God than Job did. He didn't even have the Scripture, for one thing. So I had even more grounds than he did for concluding that God knew everything and could do anything in accord with His nature. I certainly knew enough about Him to trust Him in the things that I didn't understand, such as Deb's illness.

I also realized that there were plenty of other things in the last category, too—things that I didn't know! They say that this is an inevitable result of earning a Ph.D.—you're exposed to so many items for study that you are never able to master them all. So I had no problem believing that I was finite. In fact, I never quite understood why human beings who knew better, frequently acted as if they had unlimited knowledge. But surely there is much in the universe that we do not know.

So could I really learn from Job's experiences and apply it to our situation? That's what I wanted to know. I realized that his account was included in Scripture so I could read, learn, and implement these truths. And I knew that it all made good sense, too. But what could it do for my pain?

I was also suffering, although, granted, not on the scale that Job did. Still, I wrestled with some of the same quandaries: Would Debbie be taken from us? Why did she have to suffer like this? Why was pain my constant companion during her sickness? How was I to handle what seemed to be God's silence? Why didn't God do something about the situation? Weren't we His children? Hadn't we been trying to live for Him?

I think that we probably know more often than Job did why we suffer. Scripture helps us in this regard. We have more revelation than he did, which includes the experiences of others, like Joseph's rejection by his own family, David's persecution by his family and friends alike, and the prejudice against Daniel. We also knew about the very Son of God in the Garden of Gethsemane, Paul's physical suffering and unanswered prayer, and the persecution (and even the death) of early believers. It was comforting to see that we were not alone in our struggles.

What about our particular case? What did we know? We knew that sin affected the world and pain and suffering often resulted. We knew that God had not been silent toward us. He had clearly spoken to Debbie during her worst moment in the CAT scan, forever changing her life. I knew that I couldn't charge God with not answering our prayers, and couldn't have asked for a more clear answer. Further, He seemed to reveal to me about her cancer count going down so that we could enjoy our last week of vacation together. No, I reminded myself, I couldn't say that He had been silent.

But then again, in many other things we didn't know why we were suffering. It was in these items that Job's advice was best applied. I knew that the basis for Christianity was firm. I couldn't deny this, and even in these troubled times, this gave me great comfort. Therefore, what I knew about God was sufficient to trust Him with those questions where I didn't know the answers. I could trust Him whether or not I had an explanation for a particular situation.

So how would I **actually apply** this knowledge to the numerous circumstances when I didn't know why things happened the way they did? On these occasions, I resolved to remind myself of what I **did** know about God. This approach could take many forms. Subjects for meditation could include the attributes of God, the truth about heaven, numerous other promises of God, or other aspects of His Word.

But given the more than half dozen books that I had written on the subject of Jesus' resurrection, my thoughts almost always followed a very specific trail. It had always given me instant relief during troubled times in my past. But could it have the same results in the situation with Debbie? Or would it fail to produce the desired benefits this time?

So here's what I said many times to myself during Deb's sickness: "I'm not always sure why things are happening the way they are, but this is **still** the same world in which God raised His Son from the dead. Eternal life for believers is the result. Therefore, I can trust God that there is a good answer to this situation even if I don't know what it is. At worst, I'll see Debbie again in heaven."

So how was Job's lesson applied during Debbie's struggles? How could I build a bridge between theory and practice? Even more down to earth, what would make me relax and feel better, even when I didn't know all the answers?

I pictured a situation similar to that of Job—with me asking the "Why?" questions. What would God say to me if He came and spoke to me as He did to Job in 38:3:

> Brace yourself like a man;
> I will question you,
> and you shall answer me.

What would God ask me in a situation like this one? I knew in an instant: He would undoubtedly ask me about the resurrection, about which I had done so much research. Here's a sample of how I pictured the conversation going:

"Lord, I just can't understand why You are allowing these things to happen to my family and me. Why us, especially when Debbie is so young and all four kids are still at home?"

"I just want to ask you one thing. Did I raise my Son Jesus from the dead?"

"Well yes, certainly, Lord. But how does that help me in my current sorrow?"

"Answer me once again—you do not seem to be understanding my point. Do you really believe that I raised Jesus from the dead?"

"Sure I do, but . . . ."

"Since you know that this is a world where I raised Jesus, don't you also know that His teachings are true?"

"Yes, I've always said that would follow."

"And do you have reason to think that I am still in control of the universe?"

"Yes . . . . I think you are, Sir. I have no reason to question it."

"Then isn't it also the case that, while you don't know why you are suffering, I do?"

"Well, certainly that's true."

"And whether or not you know why Debbie is suffering, have I not chosen you two in my Son, to be with me in heaven, where you'll see her again?"

"Yes, Lord. I couldn't even imagine a more glorious truth."

"Then what remains to be asked? Since you **know** these truths, including the resurrection, shouldn't you trust me in those areas where you **don't** know all of the answers?"

(Gulp)

"Do you, then, have enough knowledge to trust me through circumstances that you do not, as yet, understand?"

"I think you've got me, Lord. Yes, I should trust you with all of my heart."

"Then review and practice these truths. Don't get sidetracked by other issues, no matter how painful. You do not have to carry the heavy burden of trying to figure everything out. I want you to trust me with all of your heart."

Granted, sometimes my questions and worries were more stubborn than this. But I learned that, in these cases, I just needed to be more forceful with myself. No matter how much I hurt or how much I might have wanted to cry out in anguish, I had to make myself focus on the factual issues alone.

I can't emphasize too much the directness of the approach: I could **not** allow myself to get sidetracked here. There were very few issues that needed to be addressed at this particular point. When I wanted to shift the discussion back to the disease or to the pain, I sometimes had to forcefully say, "Not now. This is not the time for this."

Whenever the pain felt unbearable, I would sit down, usually outside on my porch. Then I forced myself to address the questions that I thought God would ask if He were challenging me, as He did Job. I quickly discovered that I could not answer this line of reasoning. Since the facts were true, the conclusion followed.

I made myself answer each of the questions as if I were hearing them for the first time. Once again, I had to decide. Do the facts say that God raised His Son from the dead? (Yes or No?) Then, is eternal life a reality? (Yes or No?) Then, are Jesus' other teachings also true? (Yes or No?) While other issues may be important, these were sufficient for me to know that everything would work out in the end, even eternally so. I would know the answers to my questions one day. I could wait, assured that there were, indeed, answers. And best of all, Debbie would be waiting for me in heaven, all smiles, for she already knew!

Of course, this might not be the exact line of questioning that God would use with everyone. I think the examination would be tailored differently, according to our own situations. For some, the issue might be, "And didn't I already answer a major prayer request (perhaps even healing) for you last year?" (Yes or No?) Or: "Didn't I save you out of some pretty bad circumstances? (Yes or No?) Or, more like Job: "You've studied (or always appreciated) my creation. Can you explain the intricacies of my design—say, the secrets of DNA or enzyme development? (Yes or No?) Or even tougher and also like Job: "Can **you** explain to me why there is pain and suffering in the world that I created?" (Yes or No?) "Why is free will necessary?"

Even though the challenge could be different, the conclusion would be the same. If we cannot explain or even understand God's ways, on what grounds can we "second guess" Him? He created the world, raised His Son from the dead, saved us, answered our prayer(s), and prepared heaven for us. Then why can't we trust Him in our present circumstances? Why can't we at least realize that He knows more than we ever could, and that includes what has happened to us?

For me, an incredible aspect of this approach is that it is definitely not based on some blind leap of faith. At no point was Job told to believe something without a basis. God pointed him to facts in the real world, usually from the areas of biology and physics. That's pretty noteworthy in an age where science is frequently thought to oppose religious belief. And the resurrection of Jesus Christ was an historical fact. No, there was no way I could say that God had asked either Job or me to believe in a vacuum.

Once again, Job's realization is the key: **what we**

already know about God is enough for us to trust Him in those things that we don't know. Such a truth should keep us focused on the most important matters in the Christian faith. Even more so, it can free us from the burden of always having to figure out exactly what God is trying to accomplish when believers hurt.

Incidentally, even the insinuation that we have a right to know God's thoughts is ridiculous, besides violating clear biblical teachings. The facts are quite simple here: I am certainly not God. Christians would readily admit this. Then why do I insist on acting like I have a right to know all of these things?

True, it could be the almost unbearable pain we're undergoing at the time that influences us to do what we probably would not do otherwise. But this is all the more reason to make sure that our suffering falls into line. In short, **it's precisely because of the pain** that we need to apply these truths, and do so forcefully! Just like suffering often leads us to think things that we would prefer not to, so it now can help us to learn and accomplish what we need to. Do we want to gain peace, or not?

This is what Job learned. He unquestionably went through some deep waters and suffered what few others have, either before or since. He responded by charging God with treating him unjustly. But God's personal challenge brought him back forcefully to his senses. In the end, Job confessed his rebellion and acknowledged that he had charged headlong into matters that he did not understand. He also recognized that God could do all things. As a result, he knew that he could trust God to take care of the deep things of the universe, including the problem of suffering and pain.

Although I didn't suffer like Job did, I still found that his remedy would work for me, precisely in the middle of my pain. I applied his lesson very often during the four months of Debbie's sickness, and it never once failed to provide relief. Every single time I thought through what would be God's challenge to me concerning the resurrection of Jesus, I realized again that the theme of Job could answer my deepest questions about our suffering. In fact, the application even became rather easy; I didn't reach it through gritted teeth.

What, precisely, did God do for me through this practice? While I still didn't know exactly why Debbie was dying, it quickly became a moot point. Anyone who knows me and my questioning mindset would realize how revolutionary this was. But the **reason** for the suffering was inconsequential. I knew that the One who had raised His Son Jesus from the dead knew the reason why. Since I couldn't deny this, I could wait for the final answer.

Along the way, I gained something else, too. Since I was no longer tempted to even ask the "Why?" question, neither did I suffer the additional emotional pain associated with not knowing the answer, or thinking that God should have done otherwise. It is well-known that emotional suffering is worse than physical pain. I could now deal with the daily issues directly in front of me, without adding the anxiety-causing distress that comes from worrying about the extra "what-ifs" of the situation. This allowed me the tremendous blessing that, whatever else happened, I knew that God was indeed in control. And I also knew that I would again be with Debbie in heaven, and for all eternity. I could rest in this, even in the middle of the suffering. It really worked, too! The relief it provided was immeasurable. God had answered my prayers once again.

10

God Will Supply

I tried to be very observant throughout the entire ordeal with Debbie's cancer. One thing I was careful to do was to keep detailed notes concerning the lessons I had learned during our suffering. Besides the message of Job, discussed in the last chapter, I concluded that there were three other, major lessons, as well as many smaller ones. Most of the items learned also served as blessings for our family.

First, I learned that God sustains His children, even in the very worst of times. Just as He states in His Word, He will never give us more than we can handle. Paul says it so nicely: "No temptation has seized you except what is common to man. And God is faithful; he will not let you be tempted beyond what you can bear. But when you are tempted, he will also provide a way out so that you can stand up under it" (1 Corinthians 10:13).

I had observed this promise being fulfilled over and over again during our trial. Some days, things would seem to be the worst I had ever experienced. I literally didn't know how I could make it through the next moment, let alone the remainder of the day. Sometimes I just wanted to crawl off and hide. Better yet, I wanted to simply push a button or have Debbie take a pill and escape it all.

But then the very next day, unbelievably, everything had done an about-face. Once, a particularly bad day in the hospital was followed by a tough night with sleep that was repeatedly broken by nurses, medicines, and the observation of machines. Then just as abruptly, as I walked the hallway early the next morning and watched the sun rise into the summer sky, I was inexplicably buoyed. Then and there, I just knew that things would work out all right, no matter what happened. I even felt strong enough to try to encourage a woman whom I had never met, but who had just lost her mother during the night.

What a change from one day to the next! It was as if David's comment had been written directly to me: "weeping may remain for a night, but rejoicing comes in the morning" (Psalm 30:5). And I knew it was the Lord Who was giving me the strength for the victory. He hadn't chosen to heal Debbie, but He did give my family and me His grace to make it through the dilemma. Yes, healing definitely comes in different forms.

Accordingly, I also realized another, very precious truth: just as the Lord had been with Debbie throughout her struggles, providing her with a very real sense of His presence, so He would be with us, when it is our time to face death. So, too, would He be with us in any other calamities that might arise.

Therefore, I didn't need to face the unknown future

with undue anxiety. I realized quite early that ongoing death anxiety, for the believer, was in all likelihood worse than death itself. As Scripture attests, Jesus Christ came in order to "free those who all their lives were held in slavery to the fear of death" (Hebrews 2:14-15). Christians can overcome excessive fear of death and experience God's peace.

Second, I knew that heaven was real and provided another great lesson that, like Job's experience, could be immediately applied to our pain. Paul commands believers who suffer to turn their thoughts away from their immediate circumstances, even their own deaths, to the reality of eternal life. God has guaranteed eternity by raising Jesus from the dead. Therefore, while our suffering is temporal, our life in heaven never ends (2 Corinthians 4:14-18).

Scarcely could this truth be stated any more clearly and beautifully than it was:

> These troubles and sufferings of ours are, after all, quite small and won't last very long. Yet this short time of distress will result in God's richest blessing upon us forever and ever! So we do not look at what we can see right now, the troubles all around us, but we look forward to the joys in heaven which we have not yet seen. The troubles will soon be over, but the joys to come will last forever (2 Corinthians 4:17-18, LB).

One thing that is so incredible here is not only does Paul tell us to meditate on future truth, but, like Job, doing so can even reduce the level of pain, which is the immediate problem! Initially, eternal life is not only real, but its very nature should give it priority in both our thinking and our acting. The pain is also real, to be sure. But Paul's advice is appropriate **even if** the pain is not thereby lessened, because eternal life is still **ultimate** reality, **long after** the suffering has subsided. In short, heaven lasts longer and is far better than earth. We are justified in thinking ahead and planning for retirement. Why shouldn't we meditate on and plan ahead for our ultimate future in heaven?

Further, Paul's teaching **can** actually lessen the pain we suffer! A positive word from a medical doctor who informs us that we are healthy often lessens our anxiety, since the emotional factor has been removed from our other symptoms. We leave the office already feeling better because we have been soothed. Similarly, a proper perspective on the truth of eternity can shift the believer's thinking away from the problems of the immediate situation. We are given the assurance that, at least ultimately, everything will be fine (especially in eternal terms!). Therefore, meditation on heaven actually allows us to refocus our attention away from the suffering, thereby lessening the emotional component. Since our emotions frequently cause the worst pain, this element alone is worthwhile.

I often thought about this message of heaven while Debbie was sick, and it was indeed comforting. In fact, given our circumstances, I couldn't imagine a more encouraging truth than this one. As I meditated on this common New Testament theme, an even more blessed angle occurred to me.

In Matthew 6:19-24, Jesus Christ commands believers to store treasures for themselves in heaven, where it cannot be contaminated by moths, rust, or robbers. Inasmuch as people themselves can be part of our eternal treasures (Philippians 4:1), I now realized that Debbie, herself, was such a prize that I was "laying up" in glory. We had mutually influenced each other in our twenty-three years of life together, and this spiritual fruit was now preserved in heaven. Therefore, **she** could not be contaminated in any way. She was, in effect, part of a heavenly bank account that could not be stolen, corrupted, or otherwise suffer any additional pain of any kind! It gave me great peace to realize that Deb had been sent ahead of me and was now waiting for me in heaven.

So the New Testament proclamation of heaven, combined with Debbie's presence there, made it all the easier to meditate on this reality rather than on my temporal circumstances. Like the message of Job, this was a great comfort to me every time I contemplated it. I do not remember a time when either theme failed to lift me up.

The third major lesson I learned was an even deeper impression of the value and sanctity of life. In a primary sense, Debbie was my closest earthly friend and the value of her life was ever before me. Secondarily, the response to our plight by family, loved ones, and friends alike was nothing short of incredible. I guess some are disturbed by the lack of help they receive in such times. But all I could do was praise God for the overwhelming show of support on our behalf.

Relatives who sacrificed so much of their vacation and personal time to be with us, church members who brought special meals, the ministry of our church worship team, colleagues who taught classes for me so I could be home with Debbie, those who sent various gifts of other sorts, as well as loving cards and phone calls, were all witnesses of love. I couldn't see them any other way. It was as if each one had the word LOVE stamped on it in bold letters.

Through this, I learned that our burdens are not meant to be carried alone. Others want to assist us and are both capable, as well as being worthy of our trust. I learned to give up jobs that Debbie or I had always handled ourselves, and, one by one, discovered that I didn't have to worry about them any longer. This was a refreshing truth to discover.

More than physical burdens, I also shared the emotional weight that I carried, especially with those close to me or with friends who had suffered similar losses. The more someone responded, the more I would share with them. Those who not only told me that they would pray for us, but were diligent in doing so, were also appreciated.

At the same time, these friends and loved ones were also suffering. Although it hurt to relive certain episodes or details by discussing them, it was often what they wanted or needed. Strangely enough, I also noticed that repeating an incident several times made it easier for me to think about and retell it the next time. At any rate, I enjoyed being able to minister to them and return the favor they had given us. It was uplifting to me when I could encourage others who were also grieving Debbie's sickness and death. Many times, it was either Job's lesson or the message of heaven that brought the blessing, too.

After all, I mused, this mutual sharing is a crucial part of the ministry in the Body of Christ. I was able to witness firsthand the pure sacrifice that occurs when brothers and sisters in Jesus Christ surrender themselves in so many ways for the benefit of others. Isn't this at least part of what the apostle Paul had in mind when he spoke about sharing and suffering together in Christ's Body (1 Corinthians 12:26)?

While these three areas plus Job's experience were the predominant lessons that I learned, other ideas also became very meaningful to me. Once again, each of these served as independent benefits, too.

I learned to appreciate the small blessings of life, whether it be a sunny day or a smile from Debbie. Even a warm meal and a good night's sleep were special. Time with the children or a note or call from a concerned friend were also welcomed. Often I thought about the fact that Deb got sick in the summer, when I could be home with her virtually the entire time. It seemed like nothing was too small to touch me.

Another blessing was how Debbie taught me to take just one day at a time. Chiefly by her example, she showed me how **not** to worry about the future. Sometimes, I even realized that I could only take a portion of a day at a time, even just an hour or two, since there was so much uncertainty. I realized that making **each moment** count for the Lord is something that we don't seem to emphasize too much any more.

I learned more than one lesson about my emotions. On the one hand, I remembered that feelings are a gift from God and are a blessing in themselves. Even during the most painful times, I could still appreciate the fact that I had feelings at all, the good along with the bad. I even became a "hugger"—something I never was before and, to tell the truth, have not kept up too much since those days. But at the time, these expressions of love and friendship were very meaningful to me, and I needed them. Men can show emotions, too!

But on the other hand, I had to apply other lessons I had learned long before—emotions also had to be controlled. Feelings can become very unruly when left to themselves, so not all experiences were good. The kind to be avoided and corrected are the ones that come from telling ourselves untruths. These can lead to additional suffering, and of an even more painful variety. I reminded myself very often (and told others, too) that we are most harmed **not** by what happens to us, but by how we cope with it and what we tell ourselves about it.

Closely aligned with controlling our emotions, I witnessed the benefit of practicing several of the biblical disciplines. Meditation was a blessing, as well as a calming influence in my life. Familiar Scripture passages leapt to life, overflowing with special meaning that they did not before have in the same way. The Book of Psalms probably became our favorite over the summer. Debbie was always blessed by Psalms 91 and 148, no matter how often I read them. Individual texts like Psalms 3:5, 4:8, and 16:11 had a profound impact on me.

I also noticed that sharing our witness to God could be more than hounding others. It could be a very natural way to share a message during the time that it will be the most readily received. In the hospital, for example, I tried never to pass up an opportunity to mention our faith to a doctor or nurse, even if it was only in some small way. Debbie did the same, probably even more than I did. It was hard not to notice that an honest word given during genuine suffering is respected by all. It was our prayer that it would affect lives, as well.

One rather profound lesson was learning that our lives are tiered. Emergency situations make us realize that very few things that we think are crucial actually are so. The wages we earn, money in general, the size of our house, the appointments we had lined up, business interests, hobbies, or summer vacations all get tested very quickly in the light of their eternal value. This is not to say that none of these, or the myriads of other things that sometimes clutter our lives, is important. Many of these items still need to be done, but the point is that an entirely new meaning is cast over them, as well as everything else that we do. And some of our practices simply fail the test altogether.

Here I made one of many mental notes. It's good to remember, I reminded myself, to be just as serious about life's priorities when current concerns are not so pressing. The reevaluating and ordering of our lives should always be a prominent consideration. As strange as it may sound, I realized even more than I did before that sometimes the seemingly frivolous pastimes, like strictly free time with children, can be as significant as anything else.

The last of my lessons concerned my immediate family. There were a great many things to be thankful for, in spite of the sobering experience of the summer. Here I had to begin with Debbie. She had always been the consummate mother and wife. Now, in front of her family, she modeled patience, love, and many other virtues. In retrospect, I do not remember any complaints from her, in spite of her situation. There were no heart-rending pleas, and virtually no requests. Her teasing and laughter were rewarding. I was so unspeakably thankful for the almost total absence of any physical or emotional pain.

Without hesitation, I attribute the lack of pain to her experience with the Lord in the CAT scan. Especially given her past fears, her present victories were inexplicable apart from His guiding hand. Beyond just having a "head knowledge" of biblical truth, her total assurance of His love, acceptance through Jesus Christ, and absence of any fear of death were nothing short of astounding. They came as a result of the wondrous grace of her loving Lord. She responded to this realization with daily praise and a cultivation of what she termed the awesomeness of God. She had modeled not only motherhood at its finest, but also devotion to God. He was the apex of her life and it was obvious. We learned from her testimony.

The children also did remarkably well during her sickness, as well as afterwards. Beyond my concern for Deb's physical condition, the four children were my chief interest. I learned a lesson about them, too: they had been exceptionally resilient, just as Judi had predicted to me. Of course there were many painful times, due to the loss of their mother. Many tearful discussions had taken place between us. But over both the summer and the months afterward, I was amazed again and again at how well they were adjusting. During their recovery, Debbie's memory was definitely not receding into the background. We took great pains to remember her regularly.

Another welcome feature of their recovery was that they were growing spiritually, as well. Here and there I heard some questions being raised by the older ones, but these were almost exclusively very early after Debbie's death and dissipated in short amounts of time. Not that questions are bad, and I knew that they could even facilitate further growth. But I was still thankful for the brevity of this stage.

Although he definitely had more questions than the others, the chief example of spiritual growth and maturation also came from my oldest child, Robbie. Though he had trusted Jesus Christ by faith as a small child, he now dates the time of his salvation from his own experience with the Lord just several months after his mother's death. The other children also kept up their interest in spiritual things, such as reading Scripture and their enjoyment of the worship portion of our church service. I regularly noted how their mother's death had little effect on their love for the Lord. Maybe it was precisely Debbie's attitude towards her Lord that caused them to respond this way.

Last of all, it seems that I could write volumes on the effect that Debbie's death had on me. In addition to all of the many lessons and blessings outlined in this volume, her suffering has had numerous, profound influences on my own spiritual life. Having previously written a book on Christian doubt and co-authored another on death and immortality, I had now experienced the latter firsthand. Many of the realizations outlined above, both theoretical as well as practical, were gems that came from her testimony and experience.

But there was also a penetrating effect on my ministry. Even though only a few friends actually mentioned it to me, I realized fairly early that others were watching us. How would we respond? Would we recover gracefully? Could I apply the principles that I had directed others to do?

I began to be asked to speak on the topic of bereavement. Whenever I did, especially when I gave Debbie's testimony of how the Lord had changed her life, I could tell that those present were giving me perhaps more attention than I had ever seen before in an audience. It was simply obvious that people were responding to her story. I had done well over a hundred radio interviews throughout my career, but when I spoke on this subject on a very small station, I received more comments than I had ever had before.

What was the Lord telling me? Was He directing me to an additional emphasis in my speaking and writing? I have concluded that Debbie's testimony, as well as the rest of the story, including both the heartache and the blessings, should now be a regular part of my ministry. It is my deepest hope that these accounts will touch many lives, just as Debbie would have wanted. As painful as certain elements were, the experience of a humble house-wife and mother will attest, even in her death, to the awesomeness of her Lord.

I will never forget you, Debbie. I will love you forever, my love.

Epilogue

I never thought that this would happen to me—or to my family. Somehow we seem to think that death is far away, until its icy fingers reach out and close around our hearts. Sometimes the news just seems to come all of a sudden, in a rush, before we can do anything about it. Then it is too late to ignore it. We are immediately forced into an emergency mode. We think that we cannot cope.

Many readers have perhaps experienced just a bit of the roller coaster that we endured during the time of Debbie's sickness and death. Then came the aftermath. As a parent, I wondered whether or not my children would "make it" and whether I was "up to" the task of helping them through their time of bereavement, in spite of my own sorrow—the very worst I had ever encountered.

In retrospect, I never think about this portion of our lives without simply marveling that the children, in particular, have all done as well as they have. I mean this most sincerely: if there ever was an indication of God's goodness in our lives, this was it! To be such a close, tight-knit family, and then to experience something so absolutely heart-rending as this, would be to think that there would be some major fallout.

But, praise God, although there were hours of discussion and counseling with each of the children, I have not been able to detect any but the most normal reactions among them. This just makes me conclude once again that God cares intensely for His children. We witnessed a number of palpable signs that this was the case. And while some may think that this account has been overly positive, I can only respond that, except for the actual cancer and Debbie's death, the other results have produced some incredible blessings.

My mother remarked to me just recently that our healing was only possible because of God's grace, and could not be accounted for by any human effort. Knowing that hundreds of people, both in this country and beyond, were praying for us was humbling in itself. We were overwhelmed with the conviction that this was God's work.

Although we could not see it at the time, going through this period as a family undoubtedly made us much stronger, both as believers and as persons. We really hope that our experiences have made an impact in our reader's lives, too. In this, I am reminded of the words of the apostle Paul:

> Praise be to the God and Father of our Lord Jesus Christ, the Father of compassion and the God of all comfort, who comforts us in all our troubles, so that we can comfort those in any trouble with the comfort we ourselves have received from God (2 Corinthians 1:3-4).

In keeping with Paul's emphasis, all of us can benefit from the suffering of others. This does not at all mean that we now know why all of this happened to our family, for this simply is not the case. Yet it seems plain to us that God still used it both for our good, as well as for the instruction of others. This gives us another perspective from which to view it. If this had to occur, for whatever reason(s), it is far better if, as a result, lives are affected for eternity.

Debbie would have agreed. That is why I shared her testimony at her funeral. Her desire was that God would receive the glory for everything that happened in her life. Could we do less than to allow others to "look in" and see what He had done?

The message rings loudly, not only in spite of Debbie's sickness, but through it. The cancer killed her body, but it could not even begin to harm her spirit. Once assured that God loved her and was going through the sickness with her, she did not fear death. Perhaps the dearest truth to us is that we will be with her someday, never again to be separated.

Suggested Further Reading

Bayly, Joseph. *The View from a Hearse*. Elgin: David C. Cook Publishing Company, 1969.

Carlson, Paul R. *Before I Wake*. Elgin: David C. Cook Publishing Company, 1975.

Feinberg, John S. *Deceived by God? A Journey Through Suffering*. Wheaton: Crossway Books, 1997.

Hunt, Gladys M. *Don't Be Afraid to Die: A Realistic Look at Death*. Grand Rapids: Zondervan Publishing House, 1971.

Jackson, Edgar N. *For the Living*. Des Moines: The Meredith Publishing Company, 1963.

Kopp, Ruth Lewshenia with Stephen Sorenson, *Encounter with Terminal Illness*. Grand Rapids: Zondervan Publishing House, 1980.

Kreeft, Peter. *Love is Stronger than Death*. San Francisco: Ignatius Press, 1979.

Kübler-Ross, Elisabeth. *On Death and Dying*. New York: Macmillan Publishing Company Inc., 1969.

Lewis, C.S. *A Grief Observed*. New York: Bantam Books, 1976.

_____. *The Problem of Pain*. New York: The Macmillan Company, 1962.

Richards, Larry and Paul Johnson. *Death and the Caring Community: Ministering to the Terminally Ill*. Portland: Multnomah Press, 1980.

Vanauken, Sheldon. *A Severe Mercy*. New York: Bantam Books, 1977.

Vetter, Robert J. *Beyond the Exit Door*. Elgin: David C. Cook Publishing Company, 1974.

Youkey, Richard. *Happily Ever After: Coping with Terminal Illness*. Joplin: College Press Publishing Company, 1991.

About the Author

Gary R. Habermas received his B.R.E. from William Tyndale College, M.A. from the University of Detroit, D.D. from Emmanuel College, Oxford, England, and Ph.D. from Michigan State University. He has ministered in three churches, the last being the Chicago Avenue United Brethren Church in Kalamazoo, Michigan. He taught Apologetics and Philosophy at Big Sky Bible College and served as Associate Professor of Apologetics and Philosophy of Religion at William Tyndale College. From 1981 to the present he is Distinguished Professor of the Department of Philosophy and Theology (Chairman since 1988) at Liberty University in Lynchburg, Virginia. Gary is also the Director of the M.A. program in Apologetics.

Among the author's 15 books are:

In Defense of Miracles: A Comprehensive Case for God's Action in History co-edited with Doug Geivett (InterVarsity, 1997).

The Historical Jesus (College Press, 1996).

A Survey of Christian Theology (Harcourt Brace, 1996).

Prolegomena to Theology (Harcourt Brace, 1996).

Why Believe? God Exists! Rethinking the Case for God and Christianity with Terry Miethe (College Press, 1993).

Immortality: The Other Side of Death with J. Moreland (Nelson, 1992).

Dealing with Doubt (Moody, 1990).

Did Jesus Rise from the Dead? The Resurrection Debate with Antony Flew, edited by Terry Miethe (Harper and Row, 1987).

Ancient Evidence for the Life of Jesus: Historical Records of His Death and Resurrection (Nelson, 1984); retitled, *The Verdict of History: Conclusive Evidence for the Life of Jesus,* 1988.

Verdict on the Shroud: Evidence for the Death and Resurrection of Jesus Christ with Kenneth Stevenson (Servant Books, 1981; Dell Publishing, 1982); ten foreign editions.

Gary Habermas

The Resurrection of Jesus: An Apologetic (Baker, 1980; University Press of America, 1984).

Gary has published six chapters in other books plus over 100 articles in journals, magazines, and reference works.

Gary has delivered over 700 lectures, including more than 50 colleges, universities, and seminaries in the U.S. and other countries, such as Stanford University, University of Pennsylvania, Rice University, Southern Methodist University, University of Virginia, Baylor University, Michigan State University, Washington University, Louisiana State University, North Carolina State University, Western Michigan University, University of Windsor (Canada), Wycliffe Hall (Oxford), University of Moscow, University of Novosibirsk (Siberia), Trinity Evangelical Divinity School, Wheaton College, Southwestern Baptist Theological Seminary, Dallas Theological Seminary, Bethel Seminary, Western (Conservative Baptist) Seminary, Taylor University, Trinity Western University, and Southeastern Baptist Theological Seminary.